Monitoring Dietary Intakes

ILSI Monographs

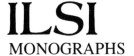

ILSI MONOGRAPHS

Sponsored by
the International
Life Sciences Institute

Ian Macdonald
Editor

Monitoring Dietary Intakes

Preface by Robert Kroes
Chairman of the Scientific Committee

Sponsored by ILSI Europe, Finnish Ministry of Trade and Industry,
Swedish National Food Administration, Food and Agricultural
Organization (FAO), World Health Organization (WHO),
European Communities

With 45 Figures

Springer-Verlag
Berlin Heidelberg New York London
Paris Tokyo Hong Kong Barcelona

Ian Macdonald, MD, DSc, FIBiol
ILSI Nutrition Co-ordinator, Emeritus Professor of Applied Physiology
Guy's Hospital Medical and Dental School, St. Thomas' Street, London SE1 9RT, UK

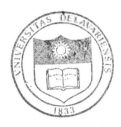

Library of Congress Cataloging-in-Publication Data
Monitoring dietary intakes / Ian Macdonald, editor ; preface by Robert
  Kroes.
     p. cm. — (ILSI monographs)
  Includes bibliographical references.
  Includes index.
  ISBN 3-540-19645-5
  1. Nutrition—Research—Methodology. 2. Nutrition surveys—
Methodology. I. Macdonald, Ian, 1921–   II. Series.
  [DNLM: 1. Nutrition. 2. Nutrition Surveys. QU 146 M744]
QP143.4.M66   1991
612.3—dc20
DNLM/DLC   90-10410
for Library of Congress

Printed on acid-free paper.

Typeset by Publishers Service of Montana, Bozeman, Montana.
Printed and bound by Edwards Brothers, Inc., Ann Arbor, Michigan.
Printed in the United States of America.

9 8 7 6 5 4 3 2 1

ISBN 3-540-19645-5 Springer-Verlag Berlin Heidelberg New York
ISBN 0-387-19645-5 Springer-Verlag New York Berlin Heidelberg

Series Foreword

The International Life Sciences Institute (ILSI), a nonprofit, public foundation, was established in 1978 to advance the sciences of nutrition, toxicology, and food safety. ILSI promotes the resolution of health and safety issues in these areas by sponsoring research, conferences, publications, and educational programs. Through ILSI's programs, scientists from government, academia, and industry unite their efforts to resolve issues of critical importance to the public.

As part of its commitment to understanding and resolving health and safety issues, ILSI is pleased to sponsor this series of monographs that consolidates new scientific knowledge, defines research needs, and provides a background for the effective application of scientific advances in toxicology and food safety.

Alex Malaspina
President
International Life Sciences Institute

Preface

We live in a changing world. The everyday, ongoing changes in people's habits and the availability of foods in the market lead to continuous changes in food consumption patterns, changes we need to understand since they play an important role in nutrition as well as toxicology.

In nutrition, food intake data provide us with the information needed to examine whether, on the one hand, these modifications are still within the limits of nutritional safety and, on the other, whether they offer the possibility of monitoring the evolution of dietary habits.

In toxicology, food intake data are used to calculate the potential intake of substances used as additives or substances that enter food as contaminants, such as pesticide residues, packaging materials, and radionuclides.

To resolve differences in food legislation, additional expert knowledge and more detailed data on food consumption and on levels of nutrients, additives and contaminants in food are necessary. For example, it is likely that certain areas of food legislation may become more liberal in an integrated Europe. Obviously, risk assessment for man will be facilitated when there are exact data on dietary intakes and on human exposure to different additives and contaminants.

Recently the Codex Committee on Food Additives and Contaminants, as well as the Codex Committee on Pesticide Residues, emphasized the importance of intake studies. According to these committees, it will be necessary to increase the number of intake studies.

Thus, adequate food intake data are a prerequisite to accurate calculations of human exposure. In the last decade numerous improvements have been made in the design and methodology of dietary surveys. But very detailed surveys are time consuming and expensive, which is why a lot of reliance is placed on population use data. These data, however, may not accurately reflect real intake.

In this volume, dietary surveys are critically assessed and their pitfalls are discussed. New data are presented that inform us especially on the actual intake of macro- and micronutrients as well as on additives and contaminants. It is interesting to see how such figures compare with established recommended dietary intakes (RDAs), acceptable daily intakes (ADIs) and maximum residue limits in foods. This comparison also provides us with better insight into margins of safety, which for some nutrients and certainly for some natural toxicants are extremely small compared with those for certain additives.

Dr. Robert J. Scheuplein, Director of the Office of Toxicological Sciences in the US Food and Drug Administration's Center for Food Safety and Applied Nutrition, said recently: "There is virtually no data worthy of the name of the daily intake of natural carcinogens. We need much better information on the identity of natural carcinogenic substances in food, the amounts present in food, and finally this information should be united with patterns of food consumption."

The objective of this volume is to provide a basis for developing better strategies for assuring food safety. It is hoped that this objective has been met.

Professor Dr. Robert Kroes
Chairman of the Scientific Committee

Contents

Contributors

The complete affiliations for all authors are given as footnotes to the opening pages of their chapters. These page numbers are given in the list below.

R. Kroes, National Institute of Public Health and Environmental Protection, The Netherlands   251

J. Kumpulainen, Food Research Institute and Central Laboratory, Finland   61

B.H. Lauer, Health and Welfare Canada   170

C. Lintas, Instituto Nazionale della Nutrizione, Rome   24

P. Lombardo, Food and Drug Administration, USA   183

A.C. Looker, National Center for Health Statistics, USA   99

K. Louekari, Ministry of Agriculture and Forestry, Helsinki   240

J.P. Mareschi, Groupe BSN, Paris   159

A. Møller, The National Food Agency of Denmark   117

J.A. Norman, Ministry of Agriculture, Fisheries and Food, London   213

Th. Ockhuizen, TN-CIVO Institutes, The Netherlands   9

E.-M. Ohlander, National Food Administration, Uppsala   191

J.A.T. Pennington, US Food and Drug Administration   3, 139

R. Rizek, US Department of Agriculture   75

Y. Saito, National Institute of Hygienic Sciences, Japan   19

C.T. Sempos, National Center for Health Statistics, USA   99

S.A. Slorach, National Food Administration, Uppsala   246

A. Turrini, Instituto Nazionale della Nutrizione, Rome   24

H.A.M.G. Vaessen, National Institute of Public Health and Environment Protection, The Netherlands   9

R.H. de Vos, TN-CIVO Institutes, The Netherlands   9

J. Wargo, Yale University, USA   75

C.E. Woteki, National Center for Health Statistics, USA   99

Part I
Methodologies of Dietary
Survey: Its Pitfalls

CHAPTER 1

Methods for Obtaining Food Consumption Information

J.A.T. Pennington[1]

The eight general methods used to assess food consumption include food disappearance data, household disappearance data, dietary histories, dietary frequencies, 24-hour recalls, food records, weighed intakes, and duplicate portions. Each method becomes refined and unique in the hands of experienced users, and innovations may be made to increase the accuracy and efficiency of data collection and evaluation. The method of choice for a particular study depends primarily upon the purposes of the study and available resources; however, other factors such as number of subjects and interviewers, abilities of subjects, and time allotted to collect dietary data may also affect the selection of the method. Memory methods (food frequencies and food recalls) are best used to access "usual intake," while actual intakes for clinical or metabolic studies might more appropriately be obtained by food records, weighed intakes, or duplicate portions. Continued improvement in all methods is needed to assess food intake more precisely and to determine the relationships of diet to health and disease.

Studies to assess dietary status and to determine the relationships between diet and health require accurate, reliable information on the foods consumed by the individuals or populations under investigation. The eight classic methods to obtain information about food intake are briefly described in Table 1.1. Innovations in some of these methods have increased the accuracy and efficiency with which the data are collected and evaluated. These innovations include computer-assisted dietary interviews, telephone interviews, on-line coding of foods, improvements in the quality and quantity of data in food composition databases, improved sampling techniques for selection of participants in "representative" surveys, and the development of "disease specific" questionnaires.

[1]Associate Director for Dietary Surveillance, Center for Food Safety and Applied Nutrition, US Food and Drug Administration, Washington, DC 20204, USA.

Table 1.1. Methods for assessing food intake

Food disappearance data – Data on national food production and food imports are corrected for food exports, food waste, food storage, and non-human food use. The results are expressed as availability of food commodities per person per day.

Household (family) disappearance data – Foods which are used in a 1-week time period in a household are corrected for food purchases, food gifts, food waste, consumption of household food by guests, and animal consumption of human foods. The results are divided by the number of persons in the household and expressed as food commodities consumed per person per day.

Dietary history (not synonymous with frequency)[a] – An open-ended questionnaire concerning food use, food preparation, portion sizes, food likes and dislikes, etc. Usually includes a 24-hour recall and/or a food frequency.

Dietary frequency (quantitative or non-quantitative) – A self-administered questionnaire consisting of a list of foods for which the respondent indicates frequency of consumption on a daily, weekly, monthly, or yearly basis. Portion sizes for the foods may be indicated.

24 hour dietary recall – An interviewer asks a subject to recall all foods eaten and portions consumed during the 24 hours of the previous day. The interviewer probes to get complete food descriptions and to help the subject remember the foods consumed.

Food record (diary) – The subject keeps a food diary for one or more days recording the names and quantities of foods consumed and when they are eaten. An interviewer usually reviews the record and probes for clarification if necessary.

Weighed/measured food intake – The subject or interviewer weighs and measures food portions prior to consumption by the subject. A written record of food descriptions and portion sizes is kept for one day or longer. Similar to the food record, except that portion sizes are more accurately measured.

Duplicate portion[b] – The subject places exact duplicates of the foods he/she consumes into a receptacle for one or more days. The foods are then homogenized and analyzed for nutrients or contaminants. A written record is usually also kept which indicates the descriptions of the foods and the quantities consumed.

---

[a]Not really a single method. Many histories include frequencies and/or recalls.
[b]Not really a method for assessing food intake, but a method for obtaining a food sample for laboratory analysis.

Unique Features of Various Methods

The food disappearance method usually relies on national data concerning food production, imports, exports, waste, and storage to make estimates of food consumed. Individual interviews are not required for this method. Food disappearance data are expressed per capita and do not allow for differentiation of food intake by age, sex, race, income, or regional groups. The household disappearance method requires at least two food inventories per household and a lengthy interview with the homemaker. The household method also does not allow evaluation of data by age or sex groups.

The questions of dietary histories are generally open-ended and are designed to elicit information for the purposes of the intended study. Dietary histories also tend to be lengthy (about 3 hours) and usually include food frequencies and/or 24-hour recalls. Complete dietary histories are rarely used in the time-conscious studies currently in progress. Food frequencies must be designated for a certain time period, e.g., the previous 3 months. They may also be designated for an earlier time in a person's life, e.g., when a 55-year-old subject was 25–35 years of age.

For 24-hour recalls, food records, weighed intakes, and duplicate portions, the number of days (and which days) to collect data must be considered and specified. More days are required to assess the usual intakes of individuals than to assess the usual intakes of groups. Also, the number of days required to obtain representative data for individuals varies according to the nutrients of concern (e.g., more days are required for vitamin A than for protein) [1]. The days for which food intake data are collected may be consecutive or distributed over time, e.g., four consecutive days or four days selected over a 3-month time period. The collection period may represent weekends and week days, although holidays are usually avoided.

The duplicate portion technique is unique in that it provides for the collection of foods for analysis of nutrients or contaminants. Thus, duplicate portion studies allow for laboratory analysis of foods, rather than calculation of nutrient content from food composition databases as the other methods do. However, in order to ascertain the foods and quantities consumed, there should be a written record of daily food intakes. Hence, the duplicate portion technique should also employ a food record or weighed intake. The duplicate portion has the distinct advantage of not requiring the matching of foods consumed to foods in food composition databases.

Method Refinement

Food consumption methods become more refined in the hands of experienced users. Modifications may be made that improve the usability, reliability, and validity of the information received. For example, food frequencies need not cover the entire diet; they may focus on foods or nutrients that are thought to be associated with specific diseases or other health effects. The 24-hour recall interviews of the Third National Health and Nutrition Examination Survey (NHANES III) are computer-assisted with on-line coding of food so that every subject gets equal treatment irrespective of the mood or disposition of the interviewer. The food consumption interviews of the United States Department of Agriculture (USDA) Nationwide Food Consumption Survey (NFCS) have default codes for foods that subjects cannot adequately remember. The default codes represent the most commonly used items in a specific food category, e.g., meat that is not further specified may default to regular ground, pan-cooked hamburger. Foods reported in the survey that are not in the database are easily added. Information about the food intake of children is obtained from parents or caregivers. The practices of these national surveys may be different from those of smaller studies where food consumption information must be obtained manually and evaluated with smaller databases.

Methodological Issues

Many papers have been published which provide information on methodological issues concerning food intake assessment. Krantzler et al. [2] have provided an annotated bibliography of 87 such papers published from 1938 to 1982. Additional papers, most of which have been published more recently, include references [3]–[8].

The usual conclusion concerning the selection of a method to assess food consumption is that the method of choice depends upon the purposes of the study and the available resources. Also to be considered are:

- The number of respondents;
- If individual or group data are needed;
- The abilities and co-operativeness of the subjects (to assess the burden that can be imposed upon the respondents);
- The staff/interviewer capabilities (to assess the burden that can be imposed upon the staff);
- The time allotted to the dietary component of the study.

The best method for assessing food consumption in a given study is usually easily identified; however, the use of the best method and the details of its usage (number of days, length of interview/questionnaire) may be restricted by the financial resources and time constraints of the study.

The type of study (population survey, epidemiology survey, clinical study, or metabolic research study) is of major concern when selecting a method for obtaining food consumption information. Most studies seek to identify usual or typical food intakes. Exceptions to this practice might be clinical or metabolic studies that attempt to correlate biochemical or physiological parameters with specific intakes of nutrients. Methods for studies not concerned with usual intake should consider weighed intakes, carefully kept food records, or duplicate portions. Methods to assess "usual" intake should rely on memory methods or methods that minimize change to usual eating habits. No method measures "true" usual intake. Comparison of the results of different methods may provide an indication of relative validity, but does not provide validation of a method. Deviation from "true intake" is due mainly to faulty memory or to changes in usual eating habits caused by the method used to assess food intake.

Memory methods include frequencies and recalls. Concerns with memory methods are that subjects may not remember all foods consumed, details about foods (e.g., cream in the coffee), or quantities consumed. Subjects may also inadvertently "remember" items not consumed. In addition, there is the problem of subject honesty. The subject may try to impress the interviewer by "improving" his/her diet, or may be unwilling to honestly report consumption of and/or amounts of some foods, especially luxury foods (desserts, snack foods, soft drinks, alcoholic beverages), if the subject views his/her intake as excessive. Likewise, the subject may inflate intake of fruit, vegetables, dairy products, meat, and grain products if the subject views his/her intake as deficient.

Non-memory methods include food records, weighed intakes, and duplicate portions. The concern with these methods is that they intrude on daily life patterns and may alter usual intake. The more intrusive the method, the more likely it is that eating habits may deviate from the norm. Record-keeping tends to decrease food intake. Food records are commonly kept for this purpose by individuals in weight-reduction programs. There may also be a tendency for the subject to eat more simply (e.g., to avoid casseroles, buffets, parties, or eating out) during the record-keeping period to reduce the tasks of recording the foods and estimating portion sizes. Honesty may also be a problem. The subject may actually improve eating habits during the record-keeping period to impress the interviewer or because the subject has become aware of faulty eating patterns through the record-keeping process. Although improvement of dietary habits is to be encouraged, if it is done only for the study period, then it is not useful for the subject or the investigator.

References

1. Karkeck JM (1987) Improving the use of dietary survey methodology. J Am Diet Assoc 87:869–871
2. Krantzler NJ, Mullen BJ, Comstock EM et al. 1982 Methods of food intake assessment — an annotated bibliography. J Nutr Educ 14:108–119
3. Carter RL, Sharbaugh CO, Stapell CA (1981) Reliability and validity of the 24-hour recall. Analysis of data from a pediatric population. J Am Diet Assoc 79:542–547
4. Hallfrisch J, Steele P, Cohen L (1982) Comparison of seven-day diet record with measured food intake of twenty-four subjects. Nutr Res 2:263–273
5. Lansky D, Brownell KD (1982) Estimates of food quantity and calories: errors in self-report among obese patients. Am J Clin Nutr 35:727–732
6. Lechtig A, Yarbrough C, Martorell R, Delgado H, Klein RE (1976) The one-day recall dietary survey: a review of its usefulness to estimate protein and calorie intake. Arch Latinoam Nutr 26:243–271
7. Liu K, Stamler K, Dyer A, McKeever J, McKeever P (1978) Statistical methods to assess and minimize the role of intra-individual variability in obscuring the relationship between dietary lipids and serum cholesterol. J Chronic Dis 31:399–418
8. Lorstad MH (1970) Food consumption surveys. Cost aspects on the precision of the estimates. Nutr Newsletter 8:21–36
9. Mahalko JR, Johnson LAK, Gallaghor SK, Milne DB (1985) Comparison of dietary histories and seven-day food records in a nutritional assessment of older adults. Am J Clin Nutr 42:542–553
10. Mullen BJ, Krantzler NJ, Grivetti LE, Schutz H, Meiselman HL (1984) Validity of a food frequency questionnaire for the determination of individual food intake. Am J Clin Nutr 39:136–143
11. Pietinen P, Tanskanen A, Tuomilehto J (1982) Assessment of sodium intake by a short dietary questionnaire. Scand J Soc Med 10:105–112
12. Posner BM, Borman CL, Morgan JL, Borden WS, Ohls JC (1982) The validity of a telephone-administered 24-hour dietary recall methodology. Am J Clin Nutr 36:546–553
13. Schucker RE (1982) Alternative approaches to classic food consumption measurement methods: telephone interviewing and market data bases. Am J Clin Nutr 35:1306–1309

14. Shapiro LR (1979) Streamlining and implementing nutritional assessment: the dietary approach. J Am Diet Assoc 75:230–237
15. Stuff JE, Garza C, Smith EOB, Nichols BL, Montandon CM (1983) A comparison of dietary methods in nutritional studies. Am J Clin Nutr 37:300–306
16. The validity of 24-hour dietary recalls. Nutr Rev 34:310–311
17. Van Leeuwen FE, De Vet HCW, Hayes RB, Van Straveren WA, West CE, Hautvast JGAJ(1983) An assessment of the relative validity of retrospective interviewing for measuring dietary intake. Am J Epidemiol 118:752–758
18. Willett WC, Sampson L, Stampfer MJ et al. (1985) Reproducibility and validity of a semiquantitative food frequency questionnaire. Am J Epidemiol 122:51–65

CHAPTER 2

The Validity of Total Diet Studies for Assessing Nutrient Intake

Th. Ockhuizen,[1] H.A.M.G. Vaessen,[2] R.H. de Vos[1] and W. van Dokkum[1]

Introduction

The nutritional quality of our diet is reflected in the balanced nutrient composition as well as in the absence, or at least the presence in acceptable low levels, of xenobiotics. Extreme nutrient intakes, either too much or too little, and excessive concentrations of contaminants and/or additives can cause major health risks.

To assess the potential risk a food-monitoring system is required. To this extent, Total Diet Studies (TDS) have been recommended on several occasions [1,2]. A TDS can be defined as a study specifically designed to establish by chemical analysis the dietary intake of food contaminants by a person consuming a typical diet. This type of study is also suitable for evaluating the macro- and micronutrient intake of (sub)populations.

The outcome of TDS is compared with available standards such as Acceptable Daily Intakes (ADIs) for additives, Provisional Tolerable Weekly Intake (PTWIs) for contaminants and Recommended Dietary Allowances (RDAs) for macro- and micronutrients. Moreover, since a monitoring system ought to include repeated sampling, the results can be compared with the previous measurements for trend analyses.

The term TDS is a collective noun for three different types of study, which are briefly described below.

Types of TDS

Market Basket Studies

Based on the known average dietary intake of the population at large, all food items which are part of the diet are purchased, resulting in a so-called market basket. It is also possible to study the diet of a population at risk instead of the

[1]TNO-CIVO Institutes, P.O. Box 360, 3700 AJ Zeist, The Netherlands.
[2]National Institute of Public Health and Environmental Protection, P.O. Box 1, 3720 BA Bilthoven, The Netherlands.

whole population. The food items are prepared according to standard household procedures and aggregated into food groups. Each food group is chemically analyzed for contaminants, additives and nutrients. A Market Basket Study (MBS) has several advantages:

1. It has a favorable cost–benefit ratio.
2. It provides an opportunity to detect trends in intake and concomitantly trends in associated risks over a time period.
3. It allows risk allocation to certain food groups.

A disadvantage is that a MBS is designed to provide insight in the "average" intake of the (sub)population and therefore does not provide information about the ranges in individual intake figures or about the risks of more extreme consumption patterns.

Individual Food Items

Based on data available from national food consumption surveys a list is compiled of the most commonly consumed food items. A good example is given by the American TDS [3], in which food items are collected in major cities of four geographic areas of the US. The foods are shipped under appropriate conditions to a central institute where the foods are, if required, prepared. Aliquots of a total of 234 composite and homogenized foods are analyzed for nutrients and contaminants.

This approach has several advantages.

1. The food sources of specific nutrients and contaminants can be identified.
2. Merging with data from the national food consumption survey renders the opportunity to estimate the intake for specific subgroups of the population, e.g. special sex and age groups.
3. The repeated sampling provides a baseline reference for determining the impact of environmental accidents on food supply (e.g. Chernobyl).

There are major disadvantages, namely variations in food preparation processes at home are not reflected, and the high costs involved.

Duplicate Portion Studies

A selected group of individuals is invited to duplicate their daily meals (after preparation), drinks and snacks. The portions are aggregated and analyzed. Duplicate Portion Studies (DPS) require the selection and co-operation of the participants. Since TDS are, among other reasons, designed to estimate the daily intake of contaminants persons can be selected who are suspected to have above average amounts of contaminants in their diet. This could be due to high food intake, e.g. in adolescents, to unusual dietary habits, e.g. vegetarians, or to environmental factors due, for instance, to living in areas where food is likely to be contaminated.

Table 2.1. Macronutrients in the Market Basket Studies of male adolescents

		1984–1986	1976–1978
Energy	(MJ/day)	13	13
Protein	(en.%[a])	14	13
Fat	(en.%)	36	39
Carbohydrates	(en.%)	46	44
Alcohol	(en.%)	4	4
Dietary fiber	(g/day)	25	18

[a]en %, percentage of energy.

The advantages of DPS are the accurate duplication of all processes that are applied to the food before consumption and the provision of direct information on the actual intake by the individuals involved. Ranges of dietary intake figures of nutrients and contaminants can be obtained. Drawbacks are first, the considerable effort asked from the participants, second, the limited time period of the study, and third, the possibility of altered food patterns while participating in the study.

Dutch Total Diet Studies

Market Basket Studies

The first MBS in the Netherlands was carried out by the TNO-CIVO Institutes in the period 1970–1978 and was followed by a second eight years later [4-6]. The dietary pattern of a group of 18-year-old males was chosen, because of their high overall intake of food and consequently their presumably high exposure to contaminants and additives. The market basket of the second study was based on food consumption data obtained from 187 adolescents with the cross-check dietary interview method. Excluding less important foods, 221 food items were purchased in the village of Zeist and aggregated into 23 food groups. Together these food items represented 98.7% of the total weight of the diet and 96.5% of the total energy. Starting in spring 1986 ten quarterly market baskets were purchased in the village of Zeist. Variations in seasonal availability of foods and in shopping areas were taken into account. A total of 36 nutrients, 114 contaminants and six additives were measured. Table 2.1 summarizes the macronutrient contents of the total diet, and Table 2.2 shows the mineral and trace element composition.

A comparison between the results of the first and second MBS yields a great deal of similarity in macronutrient composition. Only a slight increase of the percentage energy from fat and a higher daily amount of dietary fiber occurred in eight years. With respect to the micronutrients, the amounts of calcium, zinc and selenium in the total diet are adequate as compared to Provisional Dutch recommendations for male adolescents (RDA). The amounts of copper and iron can be described as marginal.

Table 2.2. Minerals and essential trace elements in the Market Basket Studies of male adolescents (mg/day)

Element	1984–1986	1976–1978	RDA[a]
Ca	1340	ND[b]	900–1200
P	2050	1860	900–1800
Fe	14	ND	15
CU	1.5	ND	1.5–3.5
Zn	14	ND	7–10
Se	0.072	0.078	0.050–0.140

[a]Provisional Dutch recommendations for male adolescents.
[b]ND, not determined.

Duplicate Portion Studies

In 1984–1985 the National Institute of Public Health and Environmental Protection repeated for the third time a DPS [7–9]. A random group of participants was selected from the population of the Utrecht area (close to Zeist). The participants were residents from rural areas, small villages, a large city (Utrecht) and several medium-sized towns. The study population reflected the total population with respect to age (18 years and older), sex and socioeconomic status. Two groups of participants (each of 56 persons) were formed and studied for one week, each in October 1984 and in March 1985. The study design required that on each day, including the weekend, eight persons had to collect a duplicate portion of all their foods and drinks. At the same time each participant completed a questionnaire. Two duplicate diets were rejected, leaving 110 duplicate diets for analyses. Laboratory tests included macro- and micronutrients as well as heavy metals, pesticides and contaminants (the results are discussed on p. 15).

Validity of Total Diet Studies

As mentioned above each type of TDS has its own set of pros and cons. Since the results of TDS are of importance for scientists as well as policy makes and may have a significant impact on future research and on political decisions, it is necessary to validate the techniques used in the study. This applies to the techniques of dietary questionnaires, sampling, shipping, preparing, analyzing and data handling. This list, which is still incomplete, holds true for all three approaches.

The present MBS was validated with respect to the nutrients in three ways.

Comparison of Nutrient Intake Data from the Dutch Market Basket Study with the National Food Consumption Survey

The food consumption pattern of the adolescents was assessed in 1982/1983 (MBS) and in 1987/1988 (National Food Composition Survey: NFCS) under different occasions, with mainly four different experimental conditions.

Table 2.3. Comparison of the results of the Market Basket Study (MBS) with the results of the National Food Consumption Survey (NFCS): food items (in 18-year-old males)

Food item	MBS (n=187) g/day	NFCS (n=63) g/day
Bread	249	233
Biscuits	48	71
Rice, macaroni etc.	32	60
Potatoes	230	169
Potato products	30	43
Leafy vegetables	61	68
Other vegetables	33	46
Soups	116	79
Root vegetables	16	37
Legume vegetable	18	8
Fresh fruits	130	88
Canned fruits/fruit juices	126	53
Meat and meat products	108	135
Poultry and eggs	33	41
Fish	9	5
Milk	316	312
Milk and dairy products	286	230
Butter, margarine, oils	64	67
Nuts	11	10
Sugar and sweets	78	85
Drinks	1257	1081
Drinking water	360	67
Miscellaneous	20	14

1. The Dutch MBS was based on the average intake of 187 18-year-old boys whereas the data from the NFCS were obtained from 63 male adolescents.
2. Dietary anamnestic techniques also differed. In the MBS the dietary history technique with cross-check was used, whereas in the NFCS participants were asked to complete a two-day food record book.
3. There is also a difference in the timespan covered by the questionnaires. In the NFCS the four seasons were covered in contrast to the MBS in which only two seasons, namely spring 1983 and autumn 1982, were covered. On the other hand in our MBS the 10 samplings were done throughout the whole year.
4. Another possible source of variation between the two methods is that food consumption patterns may have changed since the first survey. The food consumption habits of the 18-year-old males of MBS and NFCS were monitored in 1982–1983 and 1987–1988, respectively.

Table 2.3 shows a comparison of the foodgroups of both studies. Significant differences can be observed. The most striking differences are found in the group

Table 2.4. Comparison of the results of the Market Basket Study (MBS) (measured data) with the results of the National Food Consumption Survey (NFCS) (calculated data); macronutrients (in 18-year-old males)

Macronutrients		MBS ($n=187$)	NFCS ($n=63$)
Energy	(MJ)	13.3	13.5
Protein	(en.%)	13.5	12.0
Fat	(en.%)	35.3	39.4
Carbohydrates	(en.%)	46.6	47.0
Alcohol	(en.%)	4.5	1.6
Fat, saturated	(en.%)	14.6	16.1
Fat, mono-unsaturated	(en.%)	12.4	15.3
Fat, poly-unsaturated	(en.%)	4.8	6.9
Cholesterol	(mg/MJ)	26	25
P/S ratio[a]		0.33	0.43
Mono- and disaccharides	(en.%)	20.8	23.6
Dietary fiber	(g/day)	23.6	29.9

[a]P/S ratio, ratio between polyunsaturated and saturated fatty acids.

"potatoes, soups, root vegetables, fresh fruits, canned fruits/fruit juices and drinking water". It is evident that these differences in food consumption explain the differences in the intake of macronutrients (Table 2.4), minerals and trace elements (Table 2.5). When compared with the data from the NFCS, the en% fat, the P/S ratio and the amount of dietary fiber are lower in the MBS. An additional explanation for the lower en% fat in the MBS is the higher proportion of alcohol. Except for iron and copper, the intake of minerals and trace elements meets the recommended daily amounts (Table 2.5).

The outcome of the above comparison emphasizes that the results of MBS depend on the methodology used for establishing the dietary intake. Moreover, the need for up-to-date figures for the food consumption pattern is stressed.

Comparison Between the Measured and Calculated Nutrient Composition of the Dutch Market Basket Study

The measured data from the MBS were used to evaluate the validity of the Dutch Food Composition Table (NEVO-table) [10]. Table 2.6 gives the mean values of the calculated and measured intake of nutrients, together with the differences. It is obvious that the difference in dietary fiber intake between both methods is unacceptable high, namely 38%. Bread (-14.3)%, potatoes (-11.4)% and fresh and canned fruits (-7.8)% contribute most to this difference. It is concluded that, except for dietary fiber, the NEVO-table is a reliable tool for calculating the mean nutrient intake at the group level.

Table 2.5. Comparison of the results of the Market Basket Study (MBS) with the results of the National Food Consumption Survey (NFCS): minerals and trace elements (in 18-year-old males)

Element		MBS[a] (n=187)	NFCS[b] (n=63)	RDA
Ca	(mg/day)	1340	1208 (1301)[c]	900–1200
Cu	(mg/day)	1.5	1.4	1.5–3.5
Fe	(mg/day)	14	14 (14)[c]	15
Mg	(mg/day)	433	400	300–350
Se	(μg/day)	72	71	50–140
Zn	(mg/day)	14	13	7–10

[a]Analyzed data.
[b]Calculated data.
[c]Directly calculated from the total diet intake.

Comparison of Two Dutch Total Diet Studies

Since two TDS have been undertaken in the same geographical area and time period it is of interest to compare the results. It should be borne in mind, however, that first two different approaches were used, namely MBS by the TNO-CIVO Institutes and the DPS by the National Institute of Public Health and Environmental Protection. Second, the target populations differed in age, i.e. 18-year-old adolescents (MBS) versus 18–74-year-olds (DPS), and third, in the DPS alcohol is not taken into account because it is lost during freeze-drying of the samples.

In Table 2.7 the mean daily intakes of energy and macronutrients are given for both studies. Results of both studies have been normalized for 1 kg of food plus drinks. The similarity is striking. This is also true for comparison of the results for minerals and trace elements (Table 2.8). This good agreement between the

Table 2.6. Measured (Market Basket Study) and calculated (NEVO-table) nutrient intake in 18-year-old males

Nutrient	Analyzed	Calculated	Difference[a] (%)
Protein (g)	108.1	97.6	− 9.7
Fat (g)	124.8	131.9	+ 5.7
Carbohydrate (g)	364.2	394.6	+ 8.3
Dietary fiber (g)	24.5	33.8	+38.0
Calcium (mg)	1307	1422	+ 8.7
Phosphorus (mg)	2053	2103	+ 2.5
Potassium (mg)	4378	4631	+ 5.8
Iron (mg)	14.4	14.0	− 3.1
Vitamin A (mg)	1.21	1.15	− 5.0

[a]Difference = ((calculated − analyzed) : analyzed) × 100%.

Table 2.7. Comparison of the intake of macronutrients (expressed per kg food plus drinks) from the market basket and duplicate portion study (1984/1985 studies)

		CIVO-TNO market basket	RIVM duplicate portion
Energy	(kcal/kg)	868	831
Fat	(g/kg)	34	33
Protein	(g/kg)	30	31
Carbohydrate	(g/kg)	100	104

results of two different types of TDS, indicates the usefulness of both methods. The reported and observed bias of DPS (namely the underestimation of the food intake) did not apparently influence the pattern of food consumption.

Discussion

The primary aim of TDS is the assessment of the safety of the diet with respect to xenobiotics. However, since the samplings are available the nutritional adequacy of the diet can also be checked. During the Total Diet Workshop [2] it was concluded that for nutritional evaluation a minimal package of nutrients is required:

1. Macronutrients: protein, fat, carbohydrate, alcohol (from which the energy value can be calculated) and water.
2. Minerals and trace elements: Fe, Zn, Cu, Ca, Mg, Na and K.
3. Vitamins: vitamin A, B1, B2 or B6, C and folic acid.

The intake of these nutrients is compared with the RDA. Significant deviations from the RDA should be followed by relevant detailed investigations of nutritional status. Nutrient intakes below the RDA may urge the need for re-evaluation of the RDA or may stress the inadequacy of the diet for that particular nutrient in the (sub)population tested. Consistently higher values may indicate the use of supplements. In that respect DPS are of great help because they are based on individual food intakes.

In the nutritional evaluation of TDS a comparison is always made with the RDA. However, RDAs are not intended for individual guidance. Thus, inappropriate use of RDAs at an individual level could give rise to misleading conclusions.

In this chapter attention was focused on 18-year-old males because they are supposed to be highly exposed to xenobiotics. However, from a nutritional point of view other groups can be nominated as candidates for future TDS, e.g. elderly and persons with rather extreme consumption patterns. For the study of specific groups DPS are the method of choice. Analysis of all individual food items in collected market baskets (as has been done in the United States and is currently executed by the TNO-CIVO Institutes) is generally considered as a highly appropriate approach. It has the advantage that average intakes of additives, contaminants and nutrients can be evaluated for various age/sex groups and that trends can be followed. However, the high costs are a major constraint.

Table 2.8. Comparison of the intakes of minerals and trace elements (expressed per kg food plus drinks) from the market basket and duplicate portion studies 1984/1985)

Element (mg/kg)	CIVO-TNO market basket	RIVM duplicate portion
Na	1214	1099
K	1206	1283
Ca	360	377
P	566	552
Mg	120	117
Fe	4.0	4.0
Zn	3.7	3.7
Cu	0.42	0.54
Se	23.10^{-3}	19.10^{-3}

In this chapter MBS are discussed in detail and it is suggested that MBS provide useful information on the mean nutrient intake of the average diet of a particular (sub)population. The discussion of contaminants and additives is somewhat beyond the scope of the present chapter. However, MBS are also suitable to establish the daily dietary intake of these xenobiotics.

From a comparison of the intake figures of the Dutch MBS with the calculated data of the NFCS major differences have been observed. However, it can be concluded that if appropriate dietary questionnaires are used, data from NFCS may provide a solid base for TDS. The comparison of the results of the calculated and analyzed nutrient intake from the same market basket, gave support to (except for dietary fiber) the results obtained with the Dutch food composition table (NEVO-table). Finally, comparison between the results of two Dutch TDS showed striking similarities. Our overall conclusion is that MBS can provide useful and reliable information on the mean nutrient intake of the average diet of a particular (sub)population.

References

1. Anonymous (1985) Guidelines for the study of dietary intakes of chemical contaminants. WHO Offset Publication No 87, Geneva
2. Anonymous (1988) General discussion and conclusions. In: Dokkum W van, Vos RH de (eds) Dietary studies in Europe. Euronut report no 10, Wageningen pp 101–113
3. Pennington JAT (1988) Total diet studies in the USA. In: Dokkum W van, Vos RH de (eds) Dietary studies in Europe. Euronut report no 10, Wageningen, pp 51–58
4. Dokkum W van, Vos RH de, Cloughley FA et al. (1982) Food additives and food components in total diets in The Netherlands. Br J Nutr 48: 223–231
5. Vos RH de, Dokkum W van, Olthof PDA et al. (1984) Pesticides and other chemical residues in Dutch total diet samples (June 1976–July 1978). Food Chem Toxicol 22:11–21
6. Dokkum W van, Vos RH de (1988) Dietary studies in the Netherlands: Market Basket approach. In: Dokkum W van, Vos RH de (eds) Dietary studies in Europe. Euronut report no 10, Wageningen, pp 37–50

7. Vaessen HAMG, Jekel AA, Wilbers AAAM (1988) Dietary intake of polycyclic aromatic hydrocarbons. Toxicol Environ Chem 16:281–294
8. Vaessen HAMG, Kamp CG van de, Oock A van (1988) The dietary duplicate portion project 1984/1985. Performance and some results (In Dutch with summary in English). De Ware(n)-chemicus 18:30–36
9. Ellen G (1988) Dietary studies in The Netherlands: duplicate portion approach. In: Dokkum W van, Vos RH de (eds) Dietary studies in Europe. Euronut report no 10, Wageningen, 22–36
10. Erp-Baart AMJ van, Dokkum W van, Vos RH de, Wesstra JA (1989) Validity of The Netherlands Food Composition Table NEVO. Abstract Fourth Eurofoods Meeting, Uppsala

CHAPTER 3

Household Food Intake (Market Basket)

Y. Saito[1]

Introduction

In Japan, the National Institute of Hygienic Sciences is an authorizing department for the dietary intake survey of chemicals such as food contaminants and
food additives. Surveys of the intake of food pollutants have been carried out
since 1981 and of food additives since 1980 as a part of the Scientific Research
of the Ministry of Health and Welfare.

About ten municipal and prefectural institutes have been selected for each survey of food contaminant and food additive intake throughout Japan. These activities revealed the average levels of major contaminant and food additive intake.

Market Basket Study for the Determination of Dietary Intake of Pollutants

Sampling Regions and Sampling Seasons

In 1988, 11 collaborating institutes, located from northern to sourthern part of
Japan, took part in this program (Fig. 3.1), and samples were collected in summer
and autumn.

Sampling of Food

Each collaborating institute selected average food items consumed in the region
where the institute is located and estimated the food intake on the basis of the
National Nutrition Survey which classifies foods into 89 categories.

This survey, investigating the nutritional and physical status of the Japanese,
is made every year by the Ministry of Health and Welfare, Department of Public

---

[1]Division of Foods, National Institute of Hygienic Sciences, 18-1 Kamiyoga, 1-Chome,
Setogaua-Ku, Tokyo 158, Japan.

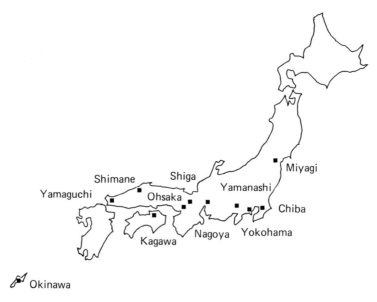

Figure 3.1. The location of the sampling site.

Health, Nutrition Section in November for three consecutive days in which 300 districts (6000 households, 21,000 persons) are chosen.

Preparation for Analyses

The 89 categories of foods are grouped into 13 sections. Drinking water (600 ml) is included as the section 14. Each food is cooked, if necessary, for table-ready consumption and analyzed for food contaminants such as organochlorinated chemicals, PCB, DDT, HCB, and organophosphorus insecticides, and heavy metals, such as mercury, cadmium, and lead, according to standard analytical methods.

The results are shown in the Tables 3.1 and 3.2.

Some Problems

There are two main problems with this method of determining dietary intake of pollutants.

1. The National Nutrition Survey which is conducted each November and forms the basis of the total diet study, excludes seasonal fluctuations in the intake of some foods. Foods produced in the summer are eaten in greater quantity in summer than in autumn and those produced in autumn are eaten much more in autumn than in summer, thus giving rise to an incorrect average intake of foods.
2. It is difficult to know the average diet of the people living in a region.

Table 3.1. Comparison of contaminant intake among food groups

	Food group														
	1	2	3	4	5	6	7	8	9	10	11	12	13	14	
Contaminants	Rice	Cereals, potatoes	Sugar, confectioneries	Fats and oil	Processed beans	Fruits	Vegetables (green)	Sea weed, vegetables	Beverages, seasonings	Fish and shellfish	Meat, egg	Milk, dairy products	Processed foods	Drinking water	Total
Total HCH	0.21[a]	0.071	0.031	0.0054	0.039	0.011	0.029	0.056	0.0063	0.024	0.096	0.051	0.041	0	0.88
Total DDT	0.057	0.02	0.0092	0.0077	0.0036	0.0031	0.049	0.0099	0	0.89	0.13	0.071	0.018	0	1.3
Dieldrin	0.055	0.0037	0.0021	0.0036	0.021	0.0085	0.012	0.061	0	0.033	0.017	0.011	0.0035	0	0.18
Hep. Epoxide	0.079	0.058	0.00078	0.011	0.0085	0.0039	0.0089	0.026	0	0.028	0.014	0.0073	0.0019	0	0.25
HCB	0	0.0052	0	0.00035	0.00024	0.0013	0.056	0.024	0.0058	0.042	0.0071	0.0073	0.0036	0	0.10
PCB	0	0	0	0.0014	0	0	0	0	0	2.48	0.22	0	0.0024	0	2.7
Malathion	0	0.44	0.038	0	0	0	0.0087	0	0	0	0	0	0.016	0	0.50
MEP	0	0.028	0	0	0	0	0	0	0	0	0.014	0.0055	0.0067	0	0.054
Diazinon	0	0	0	0	0	0	0	0	0	0	0	0	0	0	0
Pb	19	6.8	2.9	0.24	8.9	5.7	5.0	11	3.0	12	5.3	5.2	0.78	0.033	85
Cd	12	3.1	0.57	0.0018	1.4	0.30	1.7	5.6	0.96	3.5	0.66	0.30	0.28	0	29
Hg	0.63	0.20	0.050	0.029	0.02	0.045	0.058	0.04	0.0091	6.7	0.79	0.044	0.017	0	8.6
As	23	3.9	0.67	0.29	1.5	0.92	0.84	61	1.3	100	3.2	0.63	1.3	0	160

[a]Units: µg/man per day.

Table 3.2. Changes of contaminant intake

Year	Mean (μg/man/day)								Median (μg/man/day)								ADI(FAO/WHO)	
N #	1981	1982	1983	1984	1985	1986	1987	1988	1981	1982	1983	1984	1985	1986	1987	1988	μg/50 Kg	mg/Kg
	11	12	10	12	10	9	9	11	11	12	10	12	10	9	9	11		
HCH	2.9	1.8	2.6	2.1	1.2	0.89	0.69	0.88	2.4	1.8	2.21	2.24	0.94	0.87	0.55	0.48		
DDT	3.4	3.5	1.8	1.8	1.5	1.2	1.7	1.3	2.2	2.0	1.9	1.4	1.2	1.3	1.2	1.2	250	0.005
Dieldrin	0.56	0.51	0.37	0.79	0.34	0.61	0.20	0.18	0.55	0.32	0.25	0.39	0.33	0.076	0.176	0.18	5	0.0001
Hep. epoxide	0.19	0.22	0.27	0.14	0.13	0.16	0.083	0.25	0.13	0.02	0.07	0.11	0.12	0.054	0.014	0.077	25	0.0005
HCB	0.15	0.10	0.15	0.16	0.23	0.096	0.065	0.10	0.11	0.045	0.11	0.14	0.11	0.090	0.050	0.11	30[a]	0.0006[a]
PCB	3.1	2.3	2.6	2.5	2.6	1.8	2.0	2.7	2.6	1.8	2.0	1.7	1.7	2.0	1.6	1.7	250[b]	0.005[b]
Malathion	1.3	1.5	1.4	2.5	0.88	0.71	0.51	0.50	1.2	1.6	0.8	0.279	0.69	0.35	0.58	0.40	1000	0.02
MEP	0.92	2.9	1.2	0.76	0.53	0.12	1.1	0.053	0.59	1.4	1.4	0.45	0.24	0	0	0	250	0.005
Diazinon	0.44	0.03	7.9	0	0	0.048	0	0	0	0	0	0	0	0	0	0	100	0.002
Pb	54	48	71	59	48	45	48	85	37	41	81	56	40	43	38	41		
Cd	31	32	29	42	32	35	27	29	30	27	28	37	33	25	24	26		
Hg	8.4	6.9	7.9	9.3	9.7	10	11	8.6	6.6	6.8	8.7	8.8	9.9	8.5	10	8.8		
As	170	150	160	120	220	170	220	160	170	150	160	120	150	140	150	150		

[a]Withdrawn.
[b]Japanese standard.

Determination of Dietary Intake of Food Additives

The following three methods were carried out to estimate food additive intake:

1. Daily intakes of each food additive were calculated from their concentration in the foods and the food intake in the National Nutrition Survey.
2. Estimation of food additive intake was made by analyzing the food additives in the diet made from a 7-day menu.
3. The market basket method was used to determine the food additive intake in the processed foods (180 food items) which were divided into eight groups. Among the three methods, the market basket method was found to be the most practical.

Food additives were classified into Group A and Group B. Additives belonging to Group A are not found in nature, whereas those of Group B exist in nature. The average total daily intake of 50 food additives in Group A was 99.3 mg (propylene glycol, 43.0 mg; sorbic acid, 36.4 mg) whereas the average total daily intake of 140 food additives belonging to Group B was 10.0 g (glycerol, 1.27 g; glutamic acid, 1.12 g; citric acid, 0.69 g). Food additive intake of Group B in the food samples collected from nine regions throughout Japan, from Sapporo, in the north, to Kitakyushu, in the south west was found to be in the range of 9.2–11.2 g, and that of Group A was found to be in the range 53–190 mg. There are no big difference in the food additive intakes of Group B among the regions from which the food samples were collected, which may reflect the small intake of food additives. The numbers of food additives examined in this project were 50 in Group A and 140 in Group B.

The total of 347 synthetic food additives included flavors (95 items, concentration in food, < 1 ppm), and food preparation aids (not found in final food products) and other few food additives. More than 90% of synthetic food additives were analyzed in this project. There is a problem that the correct food additive intake of Group B is not obtained because of the coexistence of naturally occurring chemicals identical with those of food additives in food.

Reference

1. Ito, Y (1988) Daily intake of food additives in Japan. Ito, Y (ed) – Determination of Food Additive Residues in Food (1976–1985) – National Institute of Hygienic Sciences, Osaka Branch

CHAPTER 4

A National Food Survey. Food Balance Sheets and Other Methodologies: A Critical Overview

E. Cialfa,[1] A. Turrini,[1] and C. Lintas[1]

Introduction

The problem of the availability of food consumption data relative to one or more populations is not a new one. Because of the need in each country for a reliable data bank for intakes of nutrients and non-nutrients, for an updated evaluation of factors affecting food intakes, for nutrition education interventions and for a better approach to food policy plans, the problem of precise knowledge of food intakes becomes actual and pressing. It is well known in fact that industrialized countries have several sources of data on food intakes. They range from "Food balance sheets" (FBS) to National surveys, to more specialized and centered surveys. The methodological approaches are different as is the ability to provide better or poorer knowledge on food intake [1].

In the last years, researchers in various countries have been involved in improving methods of data survey and elaboration [2–6] and analogous efforts have been made with regard to food balance sheets [7–10].

However, the divergence still existing in the final results between data on average intakes obtained from food consumption surveys and those of National food balances (per capita disappearance data) seems to indicate that the latter should be considered approximate.

According to the FAO data (1986), the EEC countries have an "average energy intake" of 3450 Cal/cap/day, with values ranging from 3150 Cal for Portugal to 3880 (!) Cal for Belgium and Luxemburg. The EEC average lipid intake is 146 g/cap/day, with highest values for Denmark (177 g) and Belgium and Luxemburg (196 g). It is evident that such data cannot indicate the actual measure of the intake either of nutrients or foods.

At this point, the question arises whether food balance sheets can provide indications on consumptions trends, as until now it has been commonly assumed. From the FAO data it can be observed that, from 1979 to 1986, in the European countries the trend has been towards an increase in food consumption (expressed

[1]Istituto Nazionale della Nutrizione, Via Ardeatina 546, 00178 Roma, Italy.

as energy, protein and lipid). Such a trend, however, is not plausible, given the pre-existing high consumption levels, unless it is hypothesized that there is continuously increasing waste at the final consumption level.

The purpose of the study described in this chapter was to assess the value of food intake data from different sources and for different goals. To that end, data from a National food survey conducted in Italy in 1980–84 (of whose design, realization and data elaboration we are responsible) are compared with food consumption data for the same period obtained from other sources.

The National Institute of Nutrition (INN) study (from now on named "Household survey on food and nutrient intakes, INN 1980–84," or "INN survey") will be discussed in more detail. In particular, methodological problems and some relevant results will be illustrated in order to build a valid comparison with data obtained by other methods.

Household Survey on Food and Nutrient Intakes in Italy

Survey Methodology

The 1980–84 INN food survey was conducted on a sample of 10 000 households, scattered through the entire National territory. The selection of the survey units was made by random selection in three stages, with stratification of the units at the first (Region) and second (Municipality) stage to guarantee representation in relation to (a) geographical distribution and (b) class of demographic size of the municipality. The selection of the households (third stage) and their addresses were obtained through the register of voters.

Furthermore, the survey was distributed in time to take into account seasonal variations and short-period fluctuations.

The tool utilized for the survey of consumption values is the diary, where information on food behavior is also reported. Such a tool is complex and is discussed in some detail below.

In the consumption data survey, the household consumption of most of the food items for the whole period of survey (one week) was determined as the difference between the amount registered at the initial inventory, plus the additional amounts entered daily in the household (bought or received), and the quantity registered at the final inventory, minus the amounts daily given away or wasted, etc.

The amounts of food present at the beginning or the end of the survey were weighed and recorded by trained personnel (dietitians). The amounts of food bought daily or received were weighed directly by the household by means of scales provided by the INN. The amounts of food to be subtracted from consumption, because they were given away (as gifts) or wasted, were determined in the same way. The household was responsible for weighing and recording the amounts of those foods that for various reasons were not recorded at the time of the initial inventory. During the survey, the household was assisted by the dietitians to verify that all the food in the house, either consumed or not, was accurately weighed and recorded.

Actually the method adopted was a combination of a direct and an indirect survey of consumption values trying to optimize the various factors involved (personnel, households, funds and time available).

The training of the personnel and the degree of household collaboration represented a serious problem requiring considerable organizational effort. This was because such a specialized survey on such a large sample had never previously been conducted in Italy.

Given the size of the sample and consequently the very large number of consumption items, the determination of nutrient content was performed either by using official Food Composition Tables or by determining mean composition values. Consideration was also given to recipes collected for the determination of the components of cooked dishes.

Conceptual Scheme of Data

The structure of the data surveyed by the INN is schematized in Fig. 4.1. This diagram, based on the classification structures of Chen's Entity Relationship Model (as elaborated by Batini et al. [11]) (a) captures the complexity of the data surveyed, in a natural and easily understandable way [12] and (b) remains independent of the utilization context, either informatic or of a different type.

To facilitate the description of the survey structure, the scheme was subdivided into "process subschemes" relative to logically structured areas [13].*

In the brief analysis that follows reference to the subscheme is made through the titles reported in Fig. 4.1, whereas the details of the attributes relative to the individual entities and relationships are reported in Appendixes 4.1 to 4.5.

From the scheme, it can be observed that the subscheme household-person/place (Appendix 4.1) summarizes the connections between the entities family and person so allowing the transference of family information to the person and the determination of family characteristics from individual variables (number of components, composition by sex, age, education, socioeconomic level, etc.). Furthermore, as the analysis of the results will show in more detail, the geographical characteristics are variables with significant influence on food behavior.

An integral part of the subscheme person (Appendix 4.2) is the determination of those individual characteristics originating from family members which affect, or interact with, the food behavior:

1. Anthropometric characteristics
2. Type of activity
3. Diets
4. Health conditions
5. Other particular conditions

---

*The schematization proposed is only functional to the descriptive aspect and to the identification of the main applications. The subscheme concept represents in fact a bridge between basic data analysis and analysis of the processes they belong to, either informatic or not.

Figure 4.1. Conceptual
scheme.

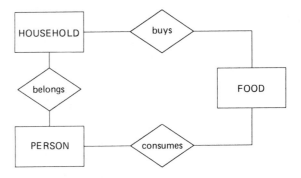

6. Role in the food organization
7. Nutrition information
8. Education

The structural characteristics of the sample basis of a food consumption analysis, were surveyed while at the same time considering their inherent motivational aspects:

1. The choice (or the rejection) of specific foods or food groups
2. Food changes taking place in recent years (subscheme household/changes-buying habits) (Appendix 4.3)

An important aspect in this type of analysis is obviously represented by the determination of the nutritive content of the food consumed. This part is represented by the subscheme food-meal (Appendix 4.4) where the different ways in which food intakes can be distributed among the various meals of the day are also shown.

All the concepts so far illustrated rotate about a central nucleus, represented in the subscheme household–person/food-meal, where all the variables essential to the determination of diet and food habits are represented (Appendix 4.5).

Such a subscheme could also be named "collection of data on food consumption" and, obviously, represents the fulcrum of any food survey. By analyzing its content, a substantial affinity of the variables assessed by the INN survey with other types of survey becomes evident, while from the standpoint of the determination of the values, several methodological differences still remain [10,14,15]. The calculation method directly affects the quality of the data obtained in a survey, which also leads to differing results.

With reference to the weekly survey period, the calculation of the per-capita daily food intake for the fth family was obtained according to formula

$$_i\bar{c}_f = (1/7) \cdot (_iC_f / \sum_{j=1}^{n_f} cp_{fj}) \tag{1}$$

$$\text{with} \quad i=1,\dots,\bar{a}; f=1,\dots,\bar{f}$$

where

$\bar{a}$ is the number of food items surveyed;
f is the number of families surveyed;
n_f is the number of components of the fth family;
$_iC_f$ is the weekly family intake of the ith food item in the fth family;
cp_{fj} is the participation coefficient of the jth person of the fth family.*

In such a formulation the calculation of the consumption in g/person/day for the entire sample is expressed as

$$_i\bar{c} = (1/7) \cdot \left(\sum_{f=1}^{\bar{f}} {_i\bar{c}_f} \cdot p_f \right) \qquad (2)$$

$$\text{with } i=1,\ldots,\bar{a};$$

where

$$p_f = \left(\sum_{j=1}^{n_f} cp_{fj} \Big/ \sum_{f=1}^{\bar{f}} \sum_{j=1}^{n_f} cp_{fj} \right)$$

$$\text{with } f=1,\ldots,\bar{f}.$$

With such an approach (a) data are standardized in relation to participation in the meals and (b) the relative weight of the meal for each person is expressed in relation to individual food habits.

----

*To determine the participation coefficient:
Step 1. Absolute weight of the tth meal of the jth person of the fth family.

$$\alpha_{fjt} = \sum_{k=1}^{\bar{k}} \alpha_{fjtk} \cdot d_{fjtk}$$

where

α_{fjtk} = weight of the kth food habit (dish) for the tth meal of the jth person belonging to the fth family
d_{fjtk} = 1 habit or 0 non-habit
k = number of codified food habits
$t = 1,\ldots,4$
Step 2. Determination of the relative weight of the tth meal of the jth person belonging to the fth family.

$$pr_{fjt} = \frac{\alpha_{fjt}}{\sum_{t=1}^{4} \alpha_{fjt}}$$

Step 3. Determination of the participation coefficient for the jth person belonging to the fth family

$$cp_{fj} = (1/7) \cdot \left(\sum_{t=1}^{4} \sum_{g=1}^{7} pr_{fjt} \cdot p_{fjtg} \right)$$

where

p_{fjtg} = 1 presence, 0 absence

indicates the presence to the tth meal of the jth person belonging to the fth family.

It has to be stressed that to render immediately comparable data relative to groups of population of different sex and age structure, "consumption units" were utilized. The methodological aspects of the determination and treatment of the INN survey data have been described in some detail to provide a basis to evaluate the type of data presented and to underline the informative potential of a food survey structured according to such methodology.

Results of the INN Survey

The first results considered are relative to the assessment of the main nutrients, expressed as amounts per day and per person (Table 4.1). The data indicate quite clearly that on average the diet dealt with here is above the RDA for energy (+15%) and especially for protein (+70%) and fat (+60%). For total carbohydrates the intake is lower than the recommendation (−18%) while at the same time showing an excess for simple sugars (+12%). The recommended intakes of micronutrients are also more or less largely covered (Fig. 4.2).

Data on nutrients and energy consumption in the different geographical areas are reported in Table 4.2. These are a traditional subdivision of Italy which differ not only in terms of economic and sociocultural factors but also historical and environmental factors.

At the present time, with its levelings and homologies, differences relative to the four geographical areas are not always very clear. However, in Italy substantial socioeconomic differences between the South and the rest of the country can still be observed. In fact, the data in Table 4.2, in particular the macronutrients, show that the intake of vegetable protein and fat, total carbohydrate and dietary fiber is higher in the South than in the other areas. The opposite is true for animal protein and fat, simple sugars, total energy and also alcohol. Anyhow, such differences are much less evident with respect to either what was expected on the basis of data from other sources or food consumption data of the recent past.

However, food consumption data are of greater speculative interest when expressed in terms of food items. In that respect, to maximize information, in the INN survey an "open" registration diary was adopted. Obviously such choice created some problems at the data treatment stage. In fact (Fig. 4.3), repeated elaborations of the food items were needed to obtain consumption data significant in strictly statistical terms but also to be utilized for the description of the phenomenon. Obviously, there are several possible aggregations of the starting items and these can be modulated according to the design of the study [16].

Data relative to 37 food items derived from more analytical tables with 138 food items (not reported here for lack of space) are shown: Average food intakes accurately depicting the Italian model of food consumption are reported in Tables 4.3 and 4.4. Omitting the analytical comments on all the food items reported in the tables, it should be observed however (Table 4.4) that the differences in food consumption of the four geographical areas are much more pronounced than those previously described expressed in terms of nutrients. This fact confirms a definite trend towards a qualitative and quantitative leveling of food intakes,

Table 4.1. Nutrient intake in Italy

	Intake (amount/ capita/day)	
	Mean	SE
Protein (g)		
Animal	59.7	0.12
Vegetable	38.1	0.07
Total	97.8	0.15
Fat (g)		
Animal	53.6	0.13
Vegetable	54.5	0.16
Total	108.1	0.22
Carbohydrate (g)	325.6	0.54
Sugar (g)	89.1	0.21
Fiber (g)	20.9	0.04
Energy (kcal)	2709	4.03
Energy from alcohol (kcal)	125	0.64
Alcohol (g)	17.8	0.09
Iron (mg)	14.9	0.03
Calcium (mg)	940.0	2.27
Thiamine (mg)	1.1	0.00
Riboflavine (mg)	1.7	0.00
Vitamin A (R.E.) (µg)	1391.5	7.73
Vitamin C (mg)	119.7	0.37
Cholesterol (mg)	347.7	1.14
Saturated fatty acid (g)	36.1	0.08
Oleic acid (g)	44.2	0.11
Linoleic acid (g)	16.3	0.07
Linolenic acid (g)	1.7	0.01
Other polyunsaturated (g)	0.5	0.01
Unsaturated fatty acid (g)	62.4	0.16

Source: Household survey on food and nutrient intakes – INN 1980–84.

expressed as nutrients, of nutrition unbalances. This trend is taking place notwithstanding food habits still being considerably different in different areas.

Comparison of Consumption Data from Different Sources

The comparison of data from different statistical sources may bring some new depths to the issue under consideration. It is clear that a comparison of data obtained by different methodologies is not entirely correct. However, its purpose

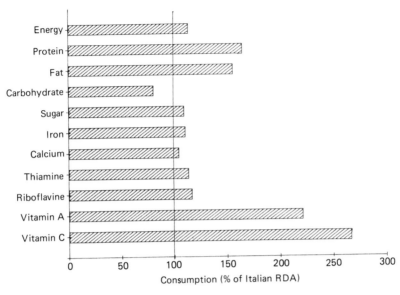

Figure 4.2. Household survey on food and nutrient intakes – INN 1980–84.

is only to verify which data can estimate real consumptions with a better approximation. In other words, whether or not an empirical comparison of information gathered by different methodologies, can provide elements of validation of the methodologies, bearing in mind different research objectives.

For the period 1980–84, some data of the INN survey were compared with analogous data of the Household Survey* conducted yearly by the Central Statistical Institute (ISTAT) [17] and with data of the National Food Balance, elaborated also by ISTAT [18] (Table 4.5). The comparison is limited to only the 15 food items included in the ISTAT surveys. It is evident from the data reported, that in most cases the consumption data of the INN survey are lower than those of the other two surveys.

In particular, the consumption values for bread, pasta, oil and wine, all typical components of the Italian diet, are considerably lower in the INN survey than in the other surveys. As regards bread, pasta and oil, the main reason may lie in the fact that in the INN survey "waste" for such food items was recorded. However, that was not always possible and consequently the INN survey also slightly over-estimates the consumption of such food items

As regards bovine meat and fish and seafood, the INN survey indicates consumption values greater than those of the ISTAT survey but closer to those of the

---

*It is a household budget survey with the object of studying levels of consumption and expenditure. The sample relative to food consumption is about 30 000 families. The recording by each family lasts ten days. Data are collected using two survey forms: the day of household expenditure by item and the summary of household expenditure. Expenditure tables contain data for 22 food items. Consumption data are presented on 15 food items.

Table 4.2. Nutrient intake in Italy in different geographical areas

	Nutrient intake (amount/capita/day)							
	North West		North East		Center		South	
	Mean	SE	Mean	SE	Mean	SE	Mean	SE
Protein (g)								
Animal	61.9	0.41	65.8	0.27	62.1	0.20	55.0	0.18
Vegetable	32.3	0.20	34.1	0.14	38.1	0.12	41.2	0.11
Total	94.2	0.54	99.9	0.34	100.1	0.26	96.2	0.23
Fat (g)								
Animal	62.9	0.46	65.4	0.31	55.4	0.22	45.1	0.17
Vegetable	44.2	0.45	52.0	0.35	54.7	0.28	58.0	0.26
Total	107.1	0.73	117.4	0.54	110.1	0.39	103.1	0.35
Carbohydrate (g)	300.5	1.82	324.5	1.29	323.3	0.98	334.3	0.82
Sugar (g)	85.6	0.64	98.4	0.55	89.0	0.39	86.3	0.32
Fiber (g)	17.9	0.12	18.3	0.09	22.0	0.07	22.1	0.06
Energy (kcal)	2585	14.23	2826	9.32	2735	7.03	2676	6.13
Energy from alcohol (kcal)	118	2.12	152	1.71	131	1.19	110	0.91
Alcohol (g)	16.8	0.30	21.8	0.24	18.7	0.17	15.8	0.13
Iron (mg)	13.8	0.09	14.8	0.06	15.6	0.05	14.8	0.04
Calcium (mg)	981.0	7.62	986.5	5.85	965.6	3.72	892.3	3.46
Thiamine (mg)	1.0	0.01	1.1	0.01	1.2	0.00	1.1	0.00
Riboflavin (mg)	1.6	0.01	1.7	0.01	1.8	0.01	1.7	0.01
Vitamin A (R.E.) (µg)	1365.4	22.66	1240.8	15.95	1501.9	15.26	1383.9	11.93
Vitamin C (mg)	104.6	1.12	103.8	0.85	138.7	0.61	117.1	0.56
Cholesterol (mg)	347.8	4.55	356.9	1.99	365.6	1.53	331.4	1.99
Saturated fatty acid (g)	41.1	0.31	41.2	0.20	37.2	0.14	32.0	0.11
Oleic acid (g)	41.7	0.35	41.7	0.24	47.3	0.21	43.6	0.18
Linoleic acid (g)	15.0	0.19	20.5	0.17	14.7	0.11	15.9	0.11
Linolenic acid (g)	1.6	0.02	1.9	0.01	1.7	0.01	1.7	0.01
Other polyunsaturated (g)	0.3	0.00	0.5	0.02	0.4	0.01	0.5	0.01
Unsaturated fatty acid (g)	58.7	0.48	64.6	0.36	64.2	0.27	61.7	0.24

Source: Household survey on food and nutrient intakes – INN 1980–84.
Data were analyzed by analysis of variance to verify the significance of the effects "geographical area" and "season." The analysis was performed according to the non-parametric Kruskal–Wallis test for K independent samples. The effect "geographical area" appears to affect significantly the difference between means, as is the case also for the effect "season."

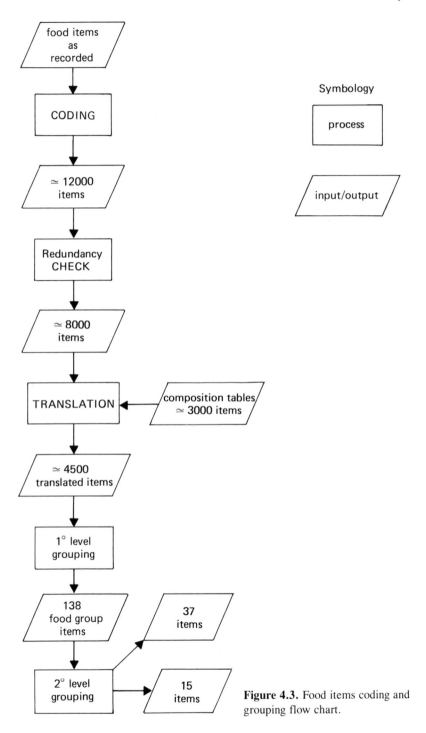

Figure 4.3. Food items coding and grouping flow chart.

Table 4.3. Food intake in Italy

	Food intake (g/capita/day)	
	Mean	SE
Bread	170.3	0.73
Pasta	79.9	0.48
Other cereal products	23.9	0.33
Rice	15.0	0.20
Legumes	30.0	0.36
Fruit	221.3	1.33
Olives	2.0	0.06
Tomatoes (for sauces)	70.5	0.67
Potatoes	50.5	0.46
Vegetables for salads	78.8	0.64
Vegetables	81.1	0.61
Bovine meat	73.8	0.47
Pig meat	7.4	0.17
Poultry and rabbit	37.9	0.39
Other meat	6.5	0.19
Offals	5.9	0.13
Sausages, sliced ham and salami	22.7	0.20
Fish and seafood	24.8	0.25
Milk	197.4	1.34
Cheese, fat <20%	14.3	0.20
Cheese, fat 20%–30%	30.7	0.26
Cheese, fat >30%	10.0	0.17
Egg	24.6	0.24
Animal fat	9.5	0.12
Vegetable oil and fat	46.1	0.26
Sauces, dressings, etc.	6.7	0.15
Sweet snacks and cookies	42.5	0.41
Snacks (salted)	1.9	0.08
Sugar and honey	30.4	0.23
Sweeteners	0.3	0.01
Coffee, tea, etc.	12.3	0.11
Mineral water	61.5	1.72
Soft drinks and juices	26.5	0.71
Beer	18.4	0.61
Wine	163.9	1.44
Liquors and spirits	2.0	0.09
Other food preparations	10.4	0.26

Source: Household survey on food and nutrient intakes – INN 1980–84.

Table 4.4. Food intake in Italy in different geographical areas

	North West Mean	North West SE	North East Mean	North East SE	Center Mean	Center SE	South Mean	South SE
Bread	135.5	1.14	139.3	0.90	163.8	0.72	193.7	0.69
Pasta	62.4	0.85	67.1	0.58	74.4	0.48	93.6	0.45
Other cereal products	25.4	0.56	33.8	0.51	30.3	0.41	19.7	0.27
Rice	24.3	0.42	21.0	0.28	12.4	0.18	12.5	0.17
Legumes	21.4	0.53	20.4	0.38	23.0	0.30	29.4	0.30
Fruit	237.7	2.58	223.0	2.12	255.0	1.53	209.2	1.19
Olives	1.0	0.05	0.8	0.05	2.4	0.07	2.6	0.06
Tomatoes (for sauces)	30.5	0.70	22.8	0.43	86.0	0.71	85.0	0.62
Potatoes	40.6	0.72	60.1	0.77	56.3	0.51	54.7	0.45
Vegetables for salads	54.3	0.84	61.5	0.75	79.8	0.66	32.3	0.32
Vegetables	76.5	1.09	82.4	1.52	97.3	0.75	81.1	0.57
Bovine meat	69.5	0.93	70.8	0.77	77.6	0.49	67.6	0.40
Pig meat	7.9	0.29	11.7	0.27	9.8	0.19	7.4	0.17
Poultry and rabbit	40.8	0.74	48.4	0.62	41.6	0.43	27.4	0.29
Other meat	5.3	0.25	3.7	0.17	6.0	0.17	6.8	0.18
Offals	7.1	0.26	6.6	0.20	5.5	0.14	6.3	0.13
Sausages, sliced ham and salami	30.9	0.41	27.3	0.35	27.5	0.23	19.0	0.16
Fish and seafood	15.6	0.45	18.2	0.30	22.7	0.25	29.3	0.24
Milk	198.7	2.52	245.9	2.16	199.9	1.29	174.1	1.12
Cheese, fat <20%	8.9	0.25	7.1	0.21	16.0	0.21	16.1	0.20
Cheese, fat 20%–30%	34.0	0.52	34.3	0.34	32.6	0.25	28.0	0.23
Cheese, fat >30%	13.2	0.30	12.2	0.25	6.6	0.12	9.2	0.14
Egg	22.8	0.83	21.9	0.30	25.5	0.23	22.9	0.34
Animal fat	14.6	0.26	15.5	0.18	8.6	0.12	5.7	0.08
Vegetable oil and fat	33.3	0.42	41.5	0.33	46.0	0.27	49.3	0.25
Sauces, dressings, etc.	8.9	0.28	9.4	0.19	6.5	0.13	4.2	0.13
Sweet snacks and cookies	52.3	0.82	51.0	0.61	45.6	0.45	29.4	0.32
Snacks (salted)	2.0	0.13	1.7	0.10	2.2	0.10	1.7	0.06
Sugar and honey	29.7	0.41	37.3	0.35	26.9	0.24	30.3	0.21
Sweeteners	0.4	0.04	0.3	0.03	0.3	0.01	0.2	0.01
Coffee, tea, etc.	13.9	0.31	14.2	0.17	13.3	0.32	11.4	0.09
Mineral water	127.5	3.96	106.5	2.68	60.8	2.01	14.3	0.92
Soft drinks and juices	27.0	1.25	29.0	1.17	17.0	0.62	18.6	0.49
Beer	13.8	0.93	16.0	0.78	12.0	0.53	14.3	0.49
Wine	150.2	2.79	191.8	2.22	171.5	1.57	144.1	1.23
Liquors and spirits	2.8	0.32	4.2	0.19	2.9	0.10	0.9	0.05
Other food preparations	17.5	0.60	15.7	0.48	14.6	0.34	6.2	0.17

Source: Household survey on food and nutrient intakes – INN 1980–84.

Table 4.5. Food consumption in Italy (1980–84): comparison of data from different sources

Products	Food consumption (g/capita/day)		
	INN[a]	ISTAT[b]	ISTAT[c]
Bread	176	203	–
Pasta	80	99	–
Bovine meat	73	65	69
Poultry	42	49	50
Other meat	31	30	27
Fish and seafood	36	22	32
Oil	44	65	53
Milk	197	224	238
Cheese	54	36	42
Egg	26	28	32
Fruit	272	225	350
Sugar	29	54	79
Coffee, tea, etc.	12	14	16
Mineral water	57	87	–
Wine	161	233	223

Statistical sources:
[a]Household survey on food and nutrient intakes, INN.
[b]Household budget surveys, ISTAT.
[c]National food balances, ISTAT.
–, Data not available.

FBS. Food balance data for bread, pasta, and mineral water are not available and data for fruit and sugar are not comparable. It is known that food balances report data expressed as basic commodities whereas consumption data surveys include several processed products containing several basic ingredients.

A comparison of the consumption of the 15 food items in the four geographical areas determined according to the INN and the ISTAT surveys is reported in Table 4.6. The previous considerations hold true also in this case. From these it can be hypothesized that the different registration methodologies, independent of the representative aspects of the samples, affect in a determining manner the control of the effective consumption levels of the different products. The fact that in the four reference areas (actually different subsamples in the two surveys compared) differences of the same order between data of the two surveys were repeated supports the hypothesis just formulated.

For this reason, further efforts should be made towards improving the quality of the observations, particularly when significant information on the consumption level of the various food items is to be provided. Furthermore, this is fundamental not only in small specialized surveys aimed at determining the intake of specific foods or food components, but also in National surveys aimed at correlating consumption data with nutritional and epidemiological evaluations.

Table 4.6. Food consumption in Italy in different geographical areas (1980–84): comparison of data from different sources

Products	Food consumption (g/capita/day)							
	North West		North East		Center		South	
	(a)	(b)	(a)	(b)	(a)	(b)	(a)	(b)
Bread	144	176	149	169	171	202	198	240
Pasta	63	76	67	69	75	103	94	128
Bovine meat	72	73	73	64	79	73	68	55
Poultry	44	47	56	49	46	60	33	45
Other meat	31	26	33	34	34	36	28	28
Fish and seafood	22	13	28	14	34	23	43	33
Oil	30	59	39	59	45	77	48	71
Milk	199	234	246	258	200	217	174	196
Cheese	56	41	54	41	56	30	53	33
Egg	26	26	25	26	29	28	26	29
Fruit	288	235	262	219	303	230	249	217
Sugar	27	56	35	58	26	52	30	52
Stimulants	13	15	13	14	13	13	11	13
Mineral water	127	143	107	110	61	73	14	40
Wine	150	257	192	263	172	263	144	183

Statistical sources:
(a), Household survey on food and nutrient intakes, INN.
(b), Household budget surveys, ISTAT.

Conclusions

The present evaluation, based on real data, about the possibility of obtaining reliable information on food consumption, supports the conclusion, beyond any doubt, that for such an objective the best source is represented by specialized food surveys. They are better in fact than either FBS or more general surveys including surveys of total consumption, either food or non-food [19].

With regard to FBS, in particular for industrialized countries, their documentary role on consumption appears to be continuously diminishing. Their limitations in providing values solely for the whole population, are well known. Also, at present, because of the considerable diversification of food consumption in industrialized countries, the increasing amount of new or processed food products, and the high levels of supply and demand (a fact leading to considerable waste), FBS can only provide an approximation, which is definitely less precise than in the past, even about average consumption levels of the population.

When consumption data, for Italy, are expressed as nutrients (Table 4.7), it can be observed than the more relevant differences are those relative to vegetable protein and fat, to carbohydrate and to alcohol. For all these products, typical of the Italian tradition, FBS data provide in fact considerably higher values. Consequently, it is in the determination of the consumption balance of the most

Table 4.7. Nutrients consumption in Italy (1980–84): comparison of data from different sources

	Amount/capita/day (mean)		% of energy	
	(a)	(b)	(a)	(b)
Protein (g)				
Animal	59.7	57.8	8.8	6.6
Vegetable	38.1	48.2	5.6	5.4
Total	97.8	106.0	14.4	12.0
Fat (g)				
Animal	53.6	66.6	17.8	17.0
Vegetable	54.5	65.6	18.1	16.8
Total	108.1	132.3	35.9	33.8
Carbohydrate (g)	325.6	449.3	45.1	47.9
Sugar (g)	89.1	137.3	12.3	14.6
Energy (kcal)	2709	3520	100.0	100.0
Energy from alcohol (kcal)	125	220	4.6	4.6

Statistical sources:
(a), Household survey on food and nutrient intakes – INN.
(b), FAO – Food Balance Sheets.

common food items (bread and pasta, cereals, oil and wine) that the intakes are considerably overestimated.

The practical result is that the per capita energy intake is more than 30% higher than the comparable average consumption obtained by the INN survey, which in turn also slightly overestimates, as previously mentioned.

It can be observed that FBS data give a consumption value that increasingly appears to be detached from reality. Being true for Italy, it can also be generalized and applied to most Western countries, with consumption data overestimated especially with regard to traditional foods. In this context, the extremely high consumption of lipid in Denmark, Belgium and Luxemburg, of animal protein in France or of vegetable protein in Greece, could also be explained.

Such limitations of FBS data used to describe the nutritional situation of a country should always be kept in mind, particularly when considering the fact that such data represent the main reference in the formulation of National and International dietary guidelines [20].

The course already undertaken by some countries of performing special surveys at regular intervals to ascertain the true consumption levels and also to validate data from other sources now appears to be mandatory, although posing serious problems in terms of organization and cost [19]. A sound nutrition policy is based on certain basic information on real consumption values or, obviously as much as possible, on their determinants.

Acknowledgments. The research in this chapter was supported by the Ministry of Agriculture and by the NRC of Italy, special grant IPRA, subproject 3. The authors wish to express their thanks to Antonella Pettinelli, Fabrizio Forlani and Marisa Capriotti for technical assistance in the preparation of the manuscript.

References

1. Jelinek F, Lindsay G (1982) Guidelines for the study of dietary intakes of contaminants. WHO: 6–19. (WHO EFP/82.36)
2. Keys A (1979) Dietary survey methods. In: Levy R, Rifkind B, Dennis B, Ernst N (eds) Nutrition, lipids and coronary heart disease. Raven Press, New York, pp 1–23
3. Bingham S, Wiggins HS, Englyst H et al. (1982) Methods and validity of dietary assessment in four Scandinavian populations. Nutr Cancer 4:23–33
4. Beaton G, Milner J, McGurie V et al. (1983) Source of variance in 24-h dietary recall data: implications for nutrient study design and interpretation. Carbohydrates sources vitamins and minerals. Am J Clin Nutr 37:986–995
5. Bingham SA (1987) The dietary assessment of individuals methods, accuracy new techniques and recommendations. pp 705–742 (Nutrition Abstracts and Reviews, Series A, vol. 57)
6. Block G, Hartman AM, Dresser GM et al (1986) A data-based approach to diet questionnaire design and testing. Am J Epidemiol 124:453–469
7. US Department of Agriculture. USDA nutrient data base for individual intake surveys. Release No. 1, Accession No PB82-138504. Springfield, VA: US Department of Commerce, National Technical Information Service
8. Manchester AC, Farrell KR (1981) Measurement and forecasting of food consumption by USDA. In: Committee on food consumption patterns of the National Research Council, assessing changing food consumption patterns. National Academy of Sciences Press, Washington, DC, pp 51–71
9. National Research Council (1984) National survey data on food consumption: uses and recommendations. National Academy of Sciences Press, Washington, DC, pp 13–30
10. Pekkarinen M (1970) Methodology in the collection of food consumption data. In: World review of nutrition and dietetics. Karger, Basel, 12:148–164
11. Batini C, De Petra G, Lenzerini M, Santucci G (1986) Il modello entità-relazione. In: La progettazione concettuale dei dati. Franco Angeli, Milano, pp 66–112
12. Hohenstein U, Gogolla M (1988) A calculus for an extended entity–relationship model incorporating arbitrary data operations and aggregate functions. In: Proceedings of the Seventh International Conference on Entity–Relationship Approach. The ER INSTITUTE, Roma, pp 1–19
13. Batini C (1989) Sviluppi metodologici per una analisi integrata dati/funzioni. In: 2° Master Users Group Meeting. GESI S.r.l., pp 30–1,36–55
14. Marr JW (1971) Individual dietary surveys: purposes and methods. In: World review of nutrition and dietetics. Karger, Basel, 13:110–139
15. Fidanza F (1984) Techniche di rilevamento delle abitudini e dei consumi alimentari. In: Fidanza F, Liguori G (eds) Nutrizione umana. Idelson, Napoli, pp 346–378
16. Cialfa E (1988) Food consumption for the evaluation of the toxicological risk. In: Lintas C, Spadoni MA (eds) Food safety and health protection. Roma, pp 241–250 (CNR IPRA, ed. Monografia No. 28)

17. ISTAT (1985) I consumi delle famiglie-anno (1984) ISTAT, Roma, pp 397–425. (Supplemento al Bollettino Mensile di Statistica, vol. 16)
18. ISTAT (1987) Annuario di Contabilità Nazionale. Roma, pp 109–125 (Series 1960–1985, vol. 15)
19. WHO (1988) Household survey data: their use in nutrition policy planning. WHO, pp 1–16 (EUR/ICP/NUT 129 OS12J)
20. James WPT in coll. with Ferro-Luzzi A, Isaksoon B, Szostak WB (1988) Healthy nutrition. WHO, Copenhagen, pp 8–13 (WHO Regional Publications, European Series, vol. 24)

Appendixes

Appendix 4.1. Subscheme Household-Person/Place

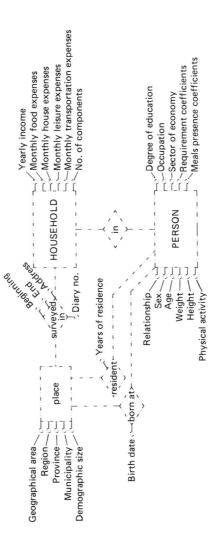

Appendix 4.2. Subscheme Person

Appendix 4.3. Subscheme Household/Changes–Buying Habits

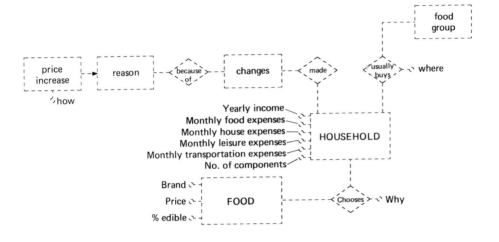

Appendix 4.4. Subscheme Food–Meal

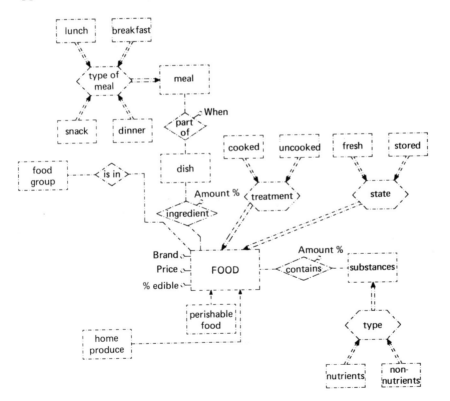

Appendix 4.5. Subscheme Household–Person/Food–Meal

44

CHAPTER 5

Estimating Human Exposure to Food Constituents

O.R. Fennema[1] and S.A. Anderson[2]

Introduction

This chapter is based on a report of the work of an Expert Panel convened by the Life Sciences Research Office of the Federation of American Societies for Experimental Biology (FASEB) under a contract from the US Food and Drug Administration.* The Expert Panel met six times during 1987 and 1988 and a report of their activities was prepared [1].

The purpose of the work was to identify and evaluate different approaches for estimating dietary exposure of humans in the US to substances in the food supply. The term "exposure" is used rather than "intake" since most of the data gathered reflects more accurately what was made available to individuals rather than what was actually consumed. Intake data are obviously preferred, but are rarely available.

Estimates of exposure, although feasible to obtain, are often lacking in quality. Nonetheless, this type of information, for reasons of practicality, provides the best, and often only, basis for evaluating the safety and nutritional adequacy of foods consumed. When estimates of human exposure to a particular substance are compared to various estimates of acceptable intake, such as acceptable daily intakes (ADI) for toxic substances or recommended dietary allowances for nutrients, the likelihood of risk associated with intake of the substance in question can be assessed.

Exposure estimates can be developed for various timespans and this has an important bearing on the details of the approach used. A single-day estimate is especially useful when ingestion of a substance is known to have an immediate effect. An estimate of "usual" exposure refers to the distribution of mean intakes of individuals over periods of several months or more. These estimates, which

[1]University of Wisconsin, Madison, WI 53706, USA.
[2]Life Sciences Research Office, Federation of American Societies for Experimental Biology, Bethesda, MD 20014, USA.
*The opinions expressed herein are those of the authors and do not necessarily reflect in full the conclusions and opinions of the Expert Panel.

are based on multiple-day food consumption data, are generally of greater usefulness than single-day estimates. Estimating usual exposure received the primary emphasis in this study.

In instances where concern lies with overconsumption of a substance because of its potential hazard to health, a meaningful objective is to estimate the 90th centile of the distribution of usual exposures (preferably extrapolated to a one-year period) for individuals in the target population. The Food and Drug Administration [2] has used this level of exposure as representative of "heavy" consumers.

Estimates of lifetime exposure to a particular substance, if accurate, would have great utility, especially in terms of evaluating carcinogenic risk. However, making accurate estimates of this kind, based on relatively short-term studies of food consumption, are almost impossible. This is true because the eating habits of any individual are not constant over time. This results from changes in age, state of health, economic status, deviation from recommended body weight, advertising and educational information, physical activity, type of foods available (geographical location; changes in products offered in the market place at a fixed location), personal habits that influence food consumption (smoking, consumption of alcoholic beverages), etc. Estimation of lifetime exposure of humans to various substances found in food was beyond the scope of this study.

Approaches Considered for Estimating Human Exposure to Substances in Food

Various approaches can be used to estimate human exposure to substances in food and a brief discussion of these approaches is useful.

Disappearance from the Marketplace

Data on the total amounts of commodities (foods or food ingredients) that "disappear" from the marketplace are available on an annual basis from government and private sources. These commodities are said to disappear because it is often not known whether the food is consumed, used for other purposes, such as feeding pets, or wasted. It is almost always correct to assume that disappearance exceeds consumption; however, a few exceptions do exist. These include intake of alcohol from fermented foods and intake of vitamins, sugars or salt added to foods that already contain these substances naturally. Annual disappearance can be divided by the corresponding annual population to obtain per capita disappearance. Per capita disappearance of foods, in turn, can be multiplied by concentration of the substance of interest to obtain a per capita mean exposure of the population to the substance. These types of data have severe limitations because they provide no indication of the distribution of exposure among individuals in the population, of the fraction of the population that did not consume the substance of interest (non-eaters), nor, as indicated earlier, of the fraction of the foods in question that were wasted or used for non-food purposes. These type of data are useful, however, for establishing trends of exposure over time and for ascertaining whether other independent estimates of exposure are realistic.

Weighing and Analysis of Foods Consumed

This approach involves, for each person being monitored, the weighing and chemical analysis of all foods consumed that contain the substance of interest. This is a near-perfect approach to determining intake of a particular substance, but suffers from the disadvantage of being so expensive that it is not feasible for use in situations involving large numbers of people. Moreover, there are indications that the act of monitoring the amount of food consumed may alter an individual's normal eating habits [3].

Market Basket Approach

This approach involves selecting foods from the marketplace that typically comprise the diets of specific age/gender groups and analyzing these foods for the constituents of interest. Based on assumptions regarding portion size, exposure estimates can be derived. The foods typically comprising the diets of the age/gender groups, and the relevant mean portion size for each food, must be derived from intake surveys. The market-basket approach has been used primarily for estimating exposure of humans to minerals and to contaminants such as pesticides; and for estimating the changes in exposure to these substances over time. Exposure data derived in this manner are of limited usefulness for determining distributions of intakes among individuals. Furthermore, this approach, as conducted by the US Food and Drug Administration (US Total Diet Study), involves a risk of not accurately representing foods that contain the specific substance of interest because only about 200 of the over 30 000 foods present in the marketplace are included in their survey.

Body Burden/Excretion

An estimate of human exposure to some dietary constituents can be made by measuring body burden (the cumulative concentration or amount of a substance in the body) or by measuring excretion of the substance of interest in the urine and/or feces. For example, exposure to ^{90}Sr from a nuclear accident or from long-term occupational exposure to radium can be determined by whole-body counting. Since these methods do not distinguish among sources of exposure, they are most useful in instances when foods are the sole or primary source of the contaminant or when the contribution of foods relative to total body burden can be estimated by other means. It should be emphasized that these measurements relate to accumulation of the test substance in the body and that accumulation depends on both absorption and retention characteristics of the body.

This approach has the disadvantage of being so time consuming and expensive that it is not feasible for use in situations involving large numbers of people.

Surveys of Consumer Intent to Purchase

This approach, which involves questioning representative groups of consumers to ascertain how often they would consume a product if it were available, is sometimes used to ascertain the likely success of new products being considered for marketing. Because the results from this approach are often unreliable, it is not a useful tool for evaluating potential exposure of humans to specific food constituents.

Food Consumption Methods

This approach involves a combination of two independently obtained types of information: (a) data on food consumption and (b) data on substance concentration. Food consumption data, in turn, consist of two major types, those collected on the basis of "quantitative daily consumption" (QDC) and those collected on the basis of "frequency of consumption" (FOC). QDC data are often collected for only a single day, although the process can be repeated to provide data for multiple days. Reference periods for FOC data are usually weeks or months, but results are generally expressed as a mean for a single day. These two similar approaches (use of QDC and FOC data) enable distributions of human exposure to the substances of interest to be estimated.

Examples of QDC databases in the US are the Nationwide Food Consumption Survey (NFCS) administered by the US Department of Agriculture, and the National Health and Nutrition Examination Survey (NHANES) administered by the National Center for Health Statistics, Department of Health and Human Services. Both of these surveys involved large, nationally representative populations and about 4500 food types. Food consumption data are collected for three non-consecutive days in the NFCS and for a single day in the NHANES.

Examples of FOC databases available for the US population are the National Household Menu Census Study administered by Market Research Corporation of America (4000 households, 14-day diary, 65 major food categories with up to 99 subcategories in each major category, frequency of consumption recorded for each household member on a daily basis) and the NPD National Eating Trends (NET) administered by the NPD Group of Marketing and Research Services, Inc. (2000 households, 14-diary, 52 food categories comprising more than 4000 different foods, frequency of consumption recorded for each household member on a daily basis).

Because food consumption data involving large population groups are available from several reliable sources and because this information can be used to estimate not only mean exposure but also the distribution of human exposure to substances in food, the FASEB Expert Panel devoted most of its attention to utilizing these types of data. The discussion that follows is confined to the use of these types of data.

Generalized Procedure for Utilizing Food Consumption Data Sources for Estimating Human Exposure to Substances in the Diet

The FASEB Expert Panel regarded the 90th centile of the distribution of usual exposures of individuals as generally representing the most meaningful type of estimate when high levels of intake are of interest. The level of exposure of the 90th centile of the population has been used by the US Food and Drug Administration to represent exposure of "heavy" consumers [2].

The following types of information are needed to estimate exposure of humans to a food substance when using the food consumption approach:

1. Foods consumed over the period of interest
2. Concentration of the substance of interest in all foods consumed by the target population
3. A procedure for evaluating validity of the results

Some difficulties associated with point (1) are the large array of foods available to the target population, the diverse consumption habits that exist in developed countries of the world and the fact that most of the consumption data available for a project of this kind are generally collected for a multiplicity of purposes and are, therefore, almost always deficient in several respects for the specific purpose intended. Some difficulties associated with point (2) are a general lack of data, poor quality or data that relate to a period that does not correspond well to that of the consumption data.

Once an exposure estimate is obtained, rigorous validation of the result (point 3) in terms of accuracy or precision is perhaps the most difficult task of all. Various approaches are available for this purpose but most that have been used in the past do not inspire confidence.

The basic procedure for making estimates of exposure using the food consumption approach is illustrated in simplified form in Fig. 5.1. Because each step within the procedure is complex, careful consideration must be given to many matters, some of which are enumerated below.

Definition of the Problem

1. *Basis for concern.* The "basis for concern" is central to defining a problem and selecting an approach for making an estimate. The nature of the concern influences whether a model is selected that overestimates or underestimates exposure. If the basis for concern is inadequate intake of a substance, then the conservative* approach is to select a model that would be unlikely to overestimate

---

*A conservative estimate is one made using assumptions that minimizes the possibility that the estimate is too low when intakes in the upper portion of the distribution are of concern, and minimizes the possibility that the estimate is too high when intakes in the lower portion of the distribution are of concern.

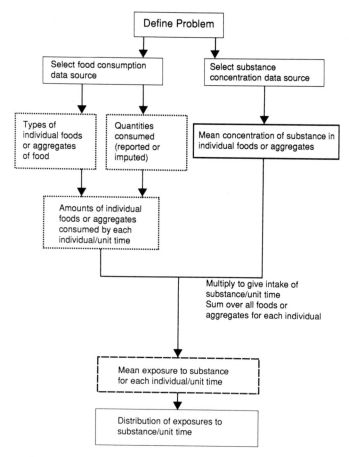

Figure 5.1. Steps for making exposure estimates based on the food consumption approach. Box with bold border: procedure to be followed for each food or aggregate of foods. Four boxes with broken borders: procedure to be followed for each individual consumer.

intake. It should be kept in mind that if inadequate intake is of concern, an error of underestimation (an estimate that is overly conservative) may result in regulatory action that is not appropriate, for example, mandating additional nutrient fortification of foods. Similarly, if the basis for concern is excess intake of a substance, the conservative approach is to select a model that is not likely to underestimate intake. In this case, an error of overestimation may lead to inappropriate regulatory action, such as limiting the concentration of an added substance in foods to levels that are lower than needed to protect public health.

2. *Population of interest.* Important sociodemographic factors should be specified. For population studies, applicable demographic descriptors might include age, race, gender, height, weight, reproductive status (pregnancy, lactation) and health status. Socioeconomic descriptors may be useful for defining subpopula-

tions of interest. In addition to sociodemographic factors, individuals in the population or subpopulation(s) might be identified as "eaters" or "non-eaters" of the substance of interest.

3. *Eating circumstances.* In addition to eating occasions at home, eating away from home will usually need to be monitored to obtain accurate estimates of human exposure to the substance of interest.

4. *Source of substance other than food.* In some instances, the substance of interest may enter the body by means other than food (e.g., water, air, dietary supplements, pharmaceuticals, cosmetics) and consideration should be given to this possibility.

Selection of a Source of Food Consumption Data

Numerous points need to be considered when selecting a food consumption database some of which are:

1. In instances where probability of excess consumption or toxicity is the basis for concern, detailed information about intakes in the upper portion of the distribution (heavy eaters) is required. In instances where likelihood of deficient consumption is the basis for concern, detailed information about intakes in the mid- to lower portion of the distribution is needed.

2. Usually it is not feasible to collect food consumption data when foods are described at the most detailed level of specificity (e.g., low calorie, chocolate chip cookies by brand name). Thus, grouping of foods is often required and this must be done with great care. When devising these food groups, the assumption is made that items within each group are consumed at fixed ratios. If this assumption is wrong, the weighted averages will be wrong. Furthermore, this averaging of food consumption that results from grouping lessens the calculated variability of food intake. Although the population mean will be unaffected [4], there will be some inaccuracy in estimates of the 90th centile of exposure. The number and types of food groups chosen also have an important bearing on whether food consumption data can be reconciled with independently collected data on substance concentration in foods.

3. User convenience is enhanced if units in the data sources selected are consistent with units that will be used for expressing the estimate.

4. It is important to assess whether the collection date for food consumption data is relevant to the time period for which an estimate is desired, and whether this date properly matches that of the substance concentration data.

5. For estimates of single-day exposure, food consumption data collected for a single day may adequately estimate mean consumption by the population provided the population sample is sufficiently large and provided the substance is widely distributed in the food supply [5–8]. However, single-day food consumption data tend to overestimate the prevalence of high or low intakes in the

distribution of intakes [9]. Single-day food consumption data are not recommended for approximation of usual exposure.

For estimates of usual exposure, either food frequency data or quantitative daily consumption data collected for multiple days are needed. Use of multiple one-day records for each individual in the survey yields a better result than use of one multiday average for each individual. Food frequency data are most useful when foods are identified with a high degree of specificity and information on portion size is collected.

6. The primary sources of error in survey-derived consumption data arise from intra-individual variation in foods consumed, sample selection, data collection and data processing. These and other erros are discussed more fully in the FASEB report. [1].

Applicability of the various types of food consumption databases for making various kinds of exposure estimates are summarized in Table 5.1.

Selection of a Source of Concentration Data

1. Information needed regarding the substance(s) of interest includes:

- Exact chemical identity
- Whether exposure to added, existing or both sources of the substance in food are of concern
- Regulatory status (may help to find sources of pertinent data)
- Routes of entry into the body such as food, air, water, dietary supplements, cosmetics, pharmaceuticals
- Bioavailability
- Extent of food specificity required (relevant to linkage problem that is discussed later)
- Variability of substance concentration within foods of interest (if available)
- Choice of foods included in the survey (inclusion of only those food sources carrying the largest concentrations of the substance of interest may, in some instances, lead to a significant underestimation of human exposure to the substance)
- Losses of the substance during processing, storage and preparation for consumption (pertinent if concentration data relate to the level of addition of the substance to the food at the time of manufacture)
- Interchangeability of the substance with other substances (if foods are grouped during the process of calculating exposure estimates, the presence of interchangeable substances can result in a gross overestimate of exposure [10]
- Date data were obtained (does this match appropriately with date when food consumption data were collected?)

Table 5.1. Potential applicability of types of food consumption data for derivation of ninetieth centile intake of a given chemical substance

| | Type of exposure estimate desired | | | |
| | Single day intake | | Usual intake | |
Type of food consumption data used	Chemical substance widely distributed	Chemical substance narrowly distributed	Chemical substance widely distributed	Chemical substance narrowly distributed
Quantitative record or recall of foods actually consumed:				
Single day	Good	Good	Poor	Poor
Multiple days	Good[a]	Good[a]	Good[b]	Good[b]
Reported frequency of usual consumption of listed foods	Poor	Poor	Good[c]	Good[c]
Market surveys of household food use[e]	Poor	Poor	Fair[d]	Poor
Disappearance data[f]	Poor	Poor	Poor	Poor
"Market basket" surveys[f]	Poor	Poor	Poor	Poor

[a]If data reported are for individual days.
[b]If number of days is sufficiently large to accept average intake as a reliable estimate of usual intake or if statistical modeling of variances is done.
[c]Potential applicability may be a function of targeting specific foods in the collection instrument.
[d]These surveys would be very good if analyzed at the level of the individual (even though serving sizes might have to be imputed), but, as usually used, the data represent disappearance into a household unit and major assumptions would need to be made about distribution within the household. The advantage of using these data is greater precision in identification of brands.
[e]Typically, 14-day food use, disaggregated to household member is reported. The underlying databases can be searched to provide intake for individual days. Identification to level of brand name is possible.
[f]Because distributions of individual food consumption cannot be obtained from disappearance data or "market basket" surveys, their primary value is as a validation measure for other estimates derived from other approaches, and for examination of time trends in exposure.
From Anderson [1]. Courtesy of LSRO, Federation of American Societies for Experimental Biology, Bethesda, MD.

2. The major sources of error in substance concentration data arise from the sampling strategy used, the type of analytical procedure chosen and how well it was executed, use of data from secondary sources, data handling procedures, and aggregation of data. A general impression of the predictability and variability of substance concentration data, as related to the type of food, is given in Table 5.2.

The matter of data aggregation deserves further comment as this common procedure can result in a large overestimate of exposure. Major supermarkets now carry about 16 000 food items. Because of the difficulty and cost of dealing with these items individually when estimating food consumption, and because composition data of the type needed is often not available for many of these foods, a common practice is to aggregate individual products into a manageable number of related groups for the purpose of calculating exposure estimates.

Table 5.2. Estimates of variability in the chemical composition of foods

Type of food substance	Type of food production or processing	Predictability of range of composition values[a]	Relative value of range (or standard deviation)
Most nutrients in canned, dried, and frozen commodities and in meat and dairy products	Controlled	Predictable	Small
Food additives	Controlled	Predictable	Small
Nutrients in recipe foods, pesticides, and GRAS substances	Controlled	Unpredictable	Large
Raw foods – normal constituents, nutrients, and natural toxicants	Uncontrolled	Predictable	Small
Contaminants	Uncontrolled	Unpredictable	Very large

[a]Predictability is based on existing knowledge of foods and substances in foods.
From Anderson [1].

Unfortunately, the food groups chosen differ in number and nature depending on the purpose of the analysis. The assumption is made that all foods in the aggregate not only contain the substance of interest, but also contain it at the same concentration. This assumption is often not true causing exposure estimates based on these food groups to be considerably overstated. If the substance is one of several more or less interchangeable substances, and it is used in only a few foods of each food group, or if a non-interchangeable substance is narrowly distributed in the food supply, the resulting overestimate of exposure can be very large, sometimes exceeding tenfold. Approaches to lessening this very severe problem have been devised for mean exposure estimates (not for 90th centile estimates) and have proven useful [10,11].

Linkage Considerations

Because it is not possible to perform chemical analyses on the actual foods consumed by participants in nationally representative surveys of food consumption, data from these surveys must be linked with separate databases for substance concentration to make exposure estimates. Compatibility between food consumption and substance concentration databases is an issue of major importance. Achieving compatibility is often the most troublesome part of the estimation process because it usually requires making unverifiable assumptions about uncertainties in the data sources or modifying one or both so that they will become compatible. Incompatibility most frequently arises because the two data sources differ in food descriptors, codes, recipes, and the nature and number of food groups used. Two options are available for dealing with database incompatibility. First, it is often possible, with a data source having numerous well-defined food groups, to combine these groups in a manner to achieve compatibility with a database having larger and fewer food groups (i.e., reducing the food groups to the least common denominator). Second, it is sometimes possible to compile a suitable substance-concentration database from several independent sources of existing data [12].

Other Considerations

The urgency with which an exposure estimate is needed, cost constraints and the desired degree of accuracy of the estimate must be considered when selecting an approach for making an exposure estimate. Unfortunately, it is not possible to know in advance all of the consequences of selecting a particular approach; thus, the selection decision must be based largely on an educated judgment regarding the anticipated consequences of the various factors.

Deriving an Estimate of Exposure to the Substance of Interest

1. When quantitative daily consumption data are used, the procedure is as follows. For each individual in the sample, the quantities of all foods consumed on single days are multiplied by the estimated substance concentration (mean value with a measure of variability should be used when possible) in each food or food group. For each person, using their data for the entire test period, a daily mean exposure estimate is determined and then a daily mean exposure estimate is calculated for the entire group of individuals in the sample. The 90th centile estimate for exposure is obtained by multiplying the 90th centile for consumption by the mean concentration of the substance of interest.

2. Alternatively, when food frequency data are used, the procedure is as follows. For each individual in the sample, the frequency of consumption of specified foods or groups of foods is multiplied by portion size (estimated or imputed) and then by the estimated substance concentration (mean with a measure of variability when possible) in the food or food group. For each person, using their data for the entire test period, a daily mean exposure estimate is determined and then a daily mean exposure estimate is calculated for the entire group of individuals in the sample. The 90th centile is derived as described above.

Validating Exposure Estimates

The process of validation should be considered an integral part of deriving usable exposure estimates. Validation should include documentation of any assumptions or calculation procedures used to assure that a conservative estimate is achieved. Either formal (statistical) or informal (comparison with other independent estimates of exposure) can be used. For the most part, the reliability of exposure estimates, as influenced by errors in food-consumption and substance-concentration databases, remains to be elucidated quantitatively. Therefore, statistical validation of currently derived exposure estimates is usually not possible; however, it is hoped that this severe shortcoming will be resolved in the near future. The approaches that can be taken to statistical validation are discussed in some detail in the FASEB report [1]. At the very least, informal validation should involve comparing the derived mean exposure estimates with means obtained or derived from other independent sources, such as market-basket data, data on body burden, manufacturing data on the substance being studied or per capita disappearance data. But even this limited validation is often difficult to accomplish in a satisfying manner.

If during validation a major discrepancy is discovered between the mean exposure estimate obtained by the food consumption approach and one or more independent estimates, it will become necessary to determine, if possible, which estimate is more accurate. This, again, is not easy to accomplish in a convincing manner. If this discrepancy remains unresolved, then the mean exposure estimate obtained, as well as the 90th centile exposure estimate, cannot be accepted with full confidence. The only way to avoid this unfortunate situation is to plan and conduct the estimation procedure with the utmost care and wisdom.

Conclusions

Procedures for estimating mean exposure of humans to substances in foods are time consuming, complex, expensive and fraught with numerous problems. These procedures become even more complex and troublesome when attempting to estimate upper or lower centiles of human exposure to substances of interest. Reasonably suitable databases for food consumption and substance concentration are seldom available, and it is rare that final estimates can be properly validated. Although difficulties in determining both concentrations of a substance in foods and consumption of foods containing the substance often render final estimates less satisfactory than desired, it is nonetheless useful, and often essential, that some estimate be made. These estimates can be achieved by using existing databases, supplemented with *ad hoc* tailor-made approaches and seasoned judgments. New technologies becoming available for the analysis of data will facilitate procedures for making exposure estimates, improve their reliability and allow reliability (accuracy and precision) to be more rigorously assessed.

Three aspects of the estimation process are especially critical. First, sound conceptualization and planning of the process must be accomplished if a satisfactory estimate of human exposure to the substance of interest is expected. Second, basic assumptions involved in arriving at the estimate should be clearly recognized, reported and included in the validation procedure. Third, a rigorous validation procedure, including estimates of variances and confidence intervals, should be a part of the estimation process. Formal statistical analysis should be completed whenever feasible. The purposes of such an analysis are to assess the accuracy and precision of the estimate and to identify those components of the estimation process that contributed most heavily to variances in the data. Informal validation techniques, although less desirable than statistical validation, are often the only type that is feasible, and they can provide checks on the reasonableness of assumptions and the final estimate.

Efforts directed to preparing databases for food consumption and substance concentration should be better co-ordinated so that available resources will result in databases that more adequately meet the needs of both governmental and industrial interests. A goal of special importance should be to improve the compatibility of food consumption and substance concentration databases. This must involve standardizing food categories that are used in both databases. Use of Universal Product Codes as food identifiers might be useful for this purpose.

Time-series forecasts of exposure to dietary components have received slight attention, despite the perception that foods and food components are changing at an ever-increasing rate. It is important that efforts be made to anticipate the likely exposure of humans to dietary components so that public policy can be formulated in an anticipatory setting rather than a reactive one.

Acknowledgments. Members of the Expert Panel that participated in the project that led to the FASEB (1988) report were: George H. Beaton, University of Toronto; Owen Fennema, University of Wisconsin; Samuel J. Fomon, University of Iowa; Richard Hall, McCormick & Co., Inc.; Clark Heath, Jr, South Carolina Department of Health and Environmental Control; James M. Lepkowski, University of Michigan; Terry L. Roe, University of Minnesota; Thomas L. Sporleder, Texas A&M University and Kent Stewart, Virginia Polytechnic Institute and State University. Their contributions to the FASEB report are acknowledged with gratitude. Support for the first author from the College of Agricultural and Life Sciences, University of Wisconsin-Madison is also acknowledged with gratitude.

References

1. Anderson SA (ed) (1988) Estimation of exposure to substances in the food supply. Report prepared for the Food and Drug Administration under Contract No. FDA 223-84-2059. Life Sciences Research Office, Federation of American Societies for Experimental Biology, Bethesda, MD
2. Food and Drug Administration (1986) Food additives permitted for direct addition to food for human consumption: aspartame. Fed Regist 51:42999–43003
3. Kim WW, Mertz W, Judd JT, Marshall MW, Kelsay JL, Prather ES (1984) Effect of making duplicate food collections on nutrient intakes calculated from diet records. Am J Clin Nutr 40:1333–1337
4. Guthrie HA, Wright HS, Krebs-Smith J, Krebs-Smith SM (1984) Assessing dietary intakes. Final report: a comparison of the food frequency with standard methods for quantifying dietary quality. US Department of Agriculture, Human Nutrition Information Service, Hyattsville, MD
5. Beaton GH, Milner J, McGuire V, Feather TE, Little JA (1983) Source of variance in 24-hour dietary recall data: implications for nutrition study design and interpretation. Carbohydrate sources, vitamins and minerals. Am J Clin Nutr 37:986–995

6. Liu K, Stamler J, Dyer A, McKeever J, McKeever P (1978) Statistical methods to assess and minimize the role of intra-individual variability in obscuring the relationship between dietary lipids and serum cholesterol. J Chron Dis 31:399–418

7. Todd KS, Hudes M, Calloway DH (1983) Food intake measurement: problems and approaches. Am J Clin Nutr 37:139–146

8. Young CM (1981) In: Assessing changing food consumption patterns. National Academy Press: Washington, DC, pp 89–118

9. Hegsted D (1972) Problems in the use and interpretation of the Recommended Dietary Allowances. Ecol Food Nutr 1:255–265

10. National Research Council (1976) Committee on GRAS List Survey – Phase III. Estimating distribution of daily intakes of certain GRAS substances. NTIS, Springfield, VA; PB299–391

11. National Research Council (1979) Committee on GRAS List Survey – Phase III. The 1977 survey of industry on the use of food additives. NTIS, Springfield, VA; PB80-113418

12. Beloian A, McDowell M (1981) Estimates of lead intakes among children up to 5 years of age, 1973–1978 and 1980. Final report. Center for Food Safety and Applied Nutrition, Food and Drug Administration, Washington, DC

Part II
Application

CHAPTER 6

Intake of Heavy Metals: Comparison of Methods

J. Kumpulainen[1]

Introduction

Due to their occurrence as environmental contaminants, relatively higher toxicity and tendency to accumulate in human organs, mercury, cadmium and lead are toxicologically the most important heavy metals.

The Joint FAO/WHO Expert Committee on Food Additives has established so-called provisional tolerable weekly intakes (PTWI) from food for these heavy metals [1]. For risk assessment, national public health authorities are required to investigate dietary intakes of heavy metals. Furthermore, monitoring of the heavy metal content of food is also an essential aspect of consumer protection, and for the facilitation of commerce. The difficulties encountered in the estimation of dietary heavy metal intakes may be divided into two main categories: (a) contamination control and analytical problems and (b) erroneous estimation of food consumption by the population group(s) studied. While the accurate estimation of food consumption is a difficulty common to all dietary intake studies, the problems associated with (a) contamination control during sampling, sample handling and analysis as well as (b) analytical methodology and (c) analytical quality control are perhaps more difficult in the case of heavy metals than with most other chemicals or elements.

The heavy metals discussed in the present paper are unevenly distributed among various food items and groups and their concentrations may differ even in comparable regions and countries. Furthermore, the concentrations of heavy metals are constantly in flux, also in foods produced in the same area, reflecting changes in various factors, such as (a) degree of industrialization, (b) number of motor vehicles, (c) degree of urbanization, (d) agricultural practice and (e) control of environmental pollution.

All of the above factors must be taken into account when planning heavy metal intake studies as well as the frequency of such investigations. Towards that goal,

[1]Food Research Institute and Central Laboratory, Agricultural Research Centre of Finland, SF-31600 Jokioinen, Finland.

the Food and Agriculture Organization of the United Nations (FAO) has published guidelines describing broad approaches for the estimation of the intakes of chemical contaminants [2]. As a complement to the above publication, the World Health Organization (WHO) has published more detailed guidelines for the study of dietary intakes of chemical contaminants [3] which are naturally applicable to studies involving heavy metals.

The purpose of this chapter is to review critically the strengths and limitations of the methods most commonly employed in dietary heavy metal intake studies, with special emphasis on practical analytical and contamination problems.

Aspects of Contamination Control, Analytical Methodology and Analytical Quality Control in Heavy Metal Intake Studies

Most foods have heavy metal concentrations in the range 1–100 ng/g dry wt. This places very high demands on the sensitivity of the analytical instrumentation to be employed in such studies. Furthermore, foods are among the most difficult matrices in terms of heavy metal analysis thus compounding the requirements of analytical methodology and instrumentation. Moreover, high environmental levels of heavy metals relative to their levels in foods make the use of dust-free rooms and clean-air hoods mandatory in dietary heavy metal studies [4].

All of the above factors contribute to the present state-of-the-art of heavy metals studies, which are far from satisfactory in general. Typically, the coefficient of variation (CV) obtained in interlaboratory comparison studies at the 10 ng/g dry wt level for any analyte is 30% or higher [5]. For heavy metals, CVs of well over 100% at this concentration level have been typical [6–8]. Recently, however, the situation has improved remarkably. This is illustrated in documents that report a decrease from 526 ng cadmium/g [7] to 1.7 ng cadmium/g [9,10] in Milk Powder and from 44 ng cadmium/g [8] to 4.9 ng cadmium/g [9,10] in Animal Muscle Reference Materials (RMs) established by the International Atomic Energy Agency (IAEA), respectively. In terms of lead content values have decreased from 267 ng/g [7] to 54 ng/g [9,10] in the IAEA Milk Powder RM. All of these recently established lower values are certified as so-called information values only.

Developments in analytical instrumentation, particularly in anodic stripping voltammetry [11,12] as well as in electrothermal atomic absorption spectrometry (ETAAS) [13,14] and the increased use of clean rooms and clean-air hoods in addition to better availability of food RMs certified for contents of heavy metal contents [6,9,15,16] are mainly responsible for the observed improvements.

However, a recently organized laboratory intercomparison study, involving laboratories specializing in trace element determinations in biological materials, on the lead content in the IAEA Animal Muscle (H-4) RM resulted in highly divergent values, therefore, its lead content could not be certified [9,10]. Moreover, a recently established [9] certified value of 160 ng lead/g dry weight in an IAEA Mixed Diet RM (commercially available) has proven too high by over 50% with a correct value being approximately 90 ng lead/g (R. Parr, IAEA, Vienna, personal communication).

These examples clearly demonstrate the complexity of the analytical problems still faced, particularly in lead analysis. It is therefore necessary to ensure the validity of an analytical method for various types of food before putting it to use. Further, it is essential to analyze samples of a RM for heavy metals together with every batch of actual samples. Naturally, the concentration level and matrix composition of a particular RM should be similar to the actual samples to be analyzed, if possible.

All of the previously mentioned problems in contamination control and in the analysis of foods for heavy metals lead to the conclusion that the risk of obtaining erroneous results is great if the number of samples with very low levels of heavy metal concentration to be analyzed is high [17,18]. Most staple foods consumed in large quantities contain very low concentrations of heavy metals being often below the limit of quantitation (LOQ) of an available analytical method [17]. If the heavy metal content of such foods is then assumed to be zero, an erroneously low intake estimate results. If, however, the content is approximated to be the same as the LOQ, an erroneously high intake estimate follows.

Attempts have been made to solve this problem by adopting the LOQ divided by two as the heavy metal content of the analyzed food item [17]. However, even in such cases the heavy metal intake estimate has been shown to result in erroneously high values [19].

However, if one intends to compose mixed market basket diets or duplicate diets, the level of heavy metal concentration is always above the limit of determination of a modern analytical method [19–21]. Further advantages of this latter approach are: (a) the considerably smaller number of samples facilitates more careful sample handling and analysis thus avoiding contaminations, and (b) the matrix composition of total diets is, from the analytical point of view, considerably easier compared to those of most staple foods and single food items, such as milk, meats, etc.

From the standpoints of analytical and contamination control it is, therefore, easier to obtain correct heavy metal intake estimates when only total diets are analyzed, and when the number of diets is as low as possible.

Evaluation of Methods to Measure Heavy Metal Intake

Introduction

In the case of heavy metals, acute food-borne poisoning is rarely a problem. The most toxic heavy metals, mercury, lead and cadmium to be dealt with here in detail, accumulate gradually in the organs. It is thus important to be able to obtain data on their average long-term intakes in order to estimate potential health risks. Therefore, if studies yielding data on long-term intakes are not possible, investigations generating data on the short-term intakes of heavy metals must be repeated on the same population at suitable intervals in order to evaluate health risks or to implement preventive measures.

There are a number of methods available for the estimation of dietary intakes of heavy metals. The best approach for a particular application depends largely on such major factors as:

1. Size of a given population
2. Availability of recent and adequate food consumption data
3. Desirability or need to measure intakes of individuals
4. Degree of literacy of a given population
5. Whether the population to be studied is a risk group
6. Whether the pattern of food consumption of a subject population group diverges widely from that of the entire population
7. Number of trained dieticians available for the study
8. Degree of sophistication of analytical instrumentation and methods of contamination control available,
9. Skills and experience of analysts,
10. The amount of funding available for the study.

As for other contaminants and specifically nutrients, the collection of food consumption data is one of the two key factors that affect the validity of the data to be obtained on the intake of heavy metals. An important factor on which the choice between various available methods is made depends upon whether data are needed on the intakes of individuals or on those of population(s).

The methods available for the study of food consumption of individual subjects are: (a) duplicate portion technique, (b) food diary with weighed intakes, (c) dietary recall, and (d) food frequency. These methods are also applicable for population studies with the exception of the duplicate portion technique, which is too laborious to be applied in large-scale population studies. In addition, national or household food disappearance methods may be employed in large-scale population studies. The above listed methods used for measuring food intake are common to all chemicals or nutrients and will not be dealt with in this context here. A detailed presentation of these methods is available [3].

Based on these methods for obtaining food consumption data, there are at present three different ways to study heavy metal intake:

1. Total diet or market basket studies
2. Calculated intake estimates based on heavy metal analyses of individual foodstuffs
3. Duplicate portion studies.

In this chapter, these methods are evaluated in light of the available literature. Due to somewhat similar approaches methods 1 and 2 will be dealt with together.

Market Basket Studies: Estimation of Intake Based on Calculation from Analyses of Individual Foodstuffs or Food Group Composites

In this method the heavy metal contents of representative samples of raw or cooked foods or food group composites are determined, thus facilitating the calculation of intakes based on food consumption figures of the population concerned. This approach may thus be employed either to study heavy metal intakes from a few foods or food groups, or total intakes of selected population groups.

The United States Food and Drug Administration (FDA) has conducted the so-called total diet study since the early 1960s. The primary aims of this study are to estimate dietary intakes of contaminants and pesticides and compare them with established intake tolerances, and to identify trends, check the effectiveness of US regulations in terms of chemicals in foods, and follow-up isolated contamination incidents.

The US total diet study approach has evolved from 82 food items originally divided into 11 food groups in 1961, to 234 analyzed food items, each representing a group of foods similar in type and nutrient content in 1984 [22]. The most significant revision took place in 1984, permitting the assessment of a greater number of age-sex groups. The food consumption data upon which the revision was based are composed of two nationwide surveys concerning approximately 50 000 participants and 5000 foods [22]. Use of the aggregation scheme thus allowed for the number of food items to be reduced to 234 instead of the 900 otherwise required to represent 95% by weight of the average US diet [22]. The food items for each market basket were collected simultaneously in three cities of one of the four geographical areas over a 4-week period. Seasonal items were collected in the appropriate city as they became available. All foods were analyzed in one laboratory after preparation according to specific instructions and combining the three like food items collected from various cities.

This study is one of the most comprehensive and probably the most carefully controlled market basket study on monitoring the intake of contaminants. This together with the fact that it is repeated at regular and frequent intervals, should ensure that it serves as a suitable case study for evaluating the validity of this methodological approach. Examination of the trends of heavy metal intake estimates (Table 6.1) shows that from 1978–1982, the estimates have been relatively constant for lead, cadmium, mercury and arsenic [23] whereas from 1982–1984 intake estimates for cadmium and lead have decreased approximately by 50% and 30%, respectively [22,23]. Although the reasons for the observed discrepancies are not completely clear, it is obvious that the change does not reflect an altered real intake, but is rather due to methodological changes introduced in 1982 [22]. The authors ascribed the differences to such factors as (a) change in the design of diets (items included and their weight representation), (b) analysis of individual food versus analysis of composites and (c) use of different analytical methods

Table 6.1. Average daily intakes (μg/day) of heavy metals in the USA in 1978–1982/84 [22,23]

Element	1978	1979	1980	1981/82	1982/84
Arsenic	45	47	48	46	45.3
Cadmium	31	32	28	28	15.4
Lead	95	82	83	57	41.3
Mercury	3	5	5	3	2.6

Table 6.2. Comparison of calculation method and chemical analysis in estimating average mineral element intakes of Finnish men [19]

Mineral element	Intake as determined by chemical analysis	Calculated intake	Difference (%)
Ca	1415 mg/day	1350 mg/day	4.6
Mg	498 mg/day	455 mg/day	8.6
Fe	19.0 mg/day	18.1 mg/day	4.7
Mn	8.0 mg/day	6.9 mg/day	13.8
Zn	15.0 mg/day	15.0 mg/day	3.3
Cu	2.0 mg/day	1.72 mg/day	14.0
Mo	110 µg/day	118 µg/day	6.8
Ni	122 µg/day	113 µg/day	9.0
Se	59 µg/day	49 µg/day	17.0
Cr	29 µg/day	33.5 µg/day	15.3
Cd	15 µg/day	24 µg/day	60
Pb	42 µg/day	135 µg/day	221
Mean ± SD			9.7 ± 5.0 (excluding Pb and Cd)

which may have affected recovery values or decreased LOQs [22]. One of the methodological problems encountered was how to treat concentrations below the LOQ. Concentrations below the LOQ were assigned a value of one-half of the LOQ. Thus, 11 foods for cadmium, eight foods for lead, 72 foods for mercury and 91 foods for arsenic belonged to this category. Moreover, 74% of the total cadmium intake estimate originated from 36 major contributing foods, while 77% of the total mercury intake estimate was derived from only four food items [22].

The role of the LOQ and the treatment of values below that limit in intake calculations is of the utmost importance in heavy metal intake studies when employing the market basket approach. An example of a study in which obviously overly low intake estimates have been obtained on cadmium and mercury intake is a study from the Netherlands [24]. In that study, eight food groups out of 12 for cadmium and mercury fell below the LOQ (5 µg/kg) and were treated as zero in the intake calculations.

The opposite way to treat values below the limit of quantitation (or detection) is to use the LOQ, or a value of half the LOQ, in the intake calculations. Even when the value of half the LOQ is used, highly erratic intake estimates may result if the LOQ is relatively high and if the number of food items analyzed is quite large [18,25]. This was clearly demonstrated in a study in which 79 total diets were composed on the basis of data on the food intake of 40 Finnish adult males. These diets were homogenized, pooled and determined for trace elements including heavy metals [19]. The analyzed intake values were then compared with intake estimates based on heavy metal determinations in 450 of the most commonly consumed foods [17]. Table 6.2 lists the intake values obtained by the above methods showing that, for elements which are relatively easy to determine accurately in foods, the agreement is usually acceptable [19,26] but for cadmium the discrepancy is 60% and for lead 221% [19]. It is possible, however, that contamination also played a role in the food preparation and analyses of the study on which the calculated intakes were based [17].

When comparing cadmium intake estimates based on the market basket method of the early 1970s and 1980s, however, a clear declining trend can be seen. In the early 1970s, typical dietary intake estimates for most countries were between 20 and 60 µg cadmium/day [23,27]. More recent values usually range from 10 to 30 µg/day for the same countries [22,28–31]. However, there is no evidence that concentrations of cadmium in cultivated soils [32] or in the food chain would have decreased during that same time period, as is the case for lead in some industrialized countries [33]. It may thus be concluded that the apparent decline in dietary cadmium intake does not reflect a change in real intake but is rather due to methodological factors, most likely improvements in analytical methodology and methods of contamination control during sample handling and analysis.

The validity of the more recent lower intake estimates is demonstrated by clinical studies in which the cadmium intake is estimated based on fecal cadmium excretion and on an average gastrointestinal cadmium absorption of 4.6% [34]. This approach resulted in an average dietary intake of cadmium of 12–20 µg/day in various US cities for adult populations [34,35]. This intake, however, is typically lower by a factor of 2 to 3 than that of most US intake estimates based on market basket methods employed in the early 1970s [23,36]. The view that the lower estimate for cadmium intake found in the recent market basket studies is more accurate is further supported by the relatively good correlation ($r=0.83$) obtained between average dietary cadmium intake in various countries and observed kidney cadmium concentration [29].

Unlike that of cadmium, the level of dietary lead intake seems to have decreased in countries where the lead content of gasoline has been reduced or removed in recent years. In the US, for example, a clear decrease in food lead content of atmospheric origin has been demonstrated, resulting in an excellent correlation ($r=0.99$) between air lead content and dietary lead intake of atmospheric origin [33]. Moreover, there is a report from Japan [37] from the early 1980s showing that the intake estimate (160 µg/day) agreed well with an estimate based on urinary and fecal lead excretion (150 µg/day).

A very useful way of checking the validity of an intake estimate in terms of contamination control and analytical quality is to analyze the food items collected from the study separately for heavy metals followed by aggregation into the major food groups analyzed for the same elements, and then to compose a final total diet which is again analyzed for the same elements. Provided that the contamination and analytical quality control are correct and that the diet has been correctly composed, the intake estimates obtained by calculation from food items, food composites or by analysis of the final diet should result in identical values.

Such an approach was undertaken in Finland by collecting 185 different food commodities so as to be representative of the average food consumption of Finns

Table 6.3. Average dietary intakes of selected elements by Finns calculated on the basis of analyses of food group composites compared with value obtained by analysis of the representative Finnish market basket diet composed of the same groups [38]

| | Intake as estimated by | | |
Element	Calculation from food groups	Analysis of final diet	Difference (%)
Fe	19.6 mg/day	20.5 mg/day	4.0
Mn	5.59 mg/day	5.48 mg/day	2.0
Zn	14.8 mg/day	16.35 mg/day	9.5
Mo	109 µg/day	107 µg/day	1.9
Ni	170 µg/day	178 µg/day	4.5
Pb	24.7 µg/day	24.0 µg/day	2.9
Cd	10.4 µg/day	12.0 µg/day	13.5
Hg	2.4 µg/day	2.3 µg/day	4.4

in 1986. The foods were divided into nine food groups, homogenized and freeze-dried. The total diet composed of the homogenates as well as the homogenates themselves were separately determined for heavy metals [38]. The agreement between the calculated and analyzed intake estimates was excellent for all of the heavy metals determined (Table 6.3). These data demonstrate that for heavy metals, even lead, a carefully controlled market basket study can result in reliable intake estimates.

Duplicate Portion Studies

By the duplicate portion technique, representative diets of individuals can be collected usually over a time span of one day to weeks, by requesting representative subjects of a target population to provide a duplicate sample of meals they have consumed during a given time period. Naturally, this method may be also applied to institutions, such as hospitals, where a trained dietician is often available. The duplicate portion technique may also be applied to the earlier mentioned food diary and weighed intake studies.

The market basket method is suitable for investigating the heavy metal intakes of large populations, but the duplicate portion method is not applicable for this type of study owing to the considerable field staff burden and costs involved. It usually takes at least two or more home visits by a dietician to educate and motivate subjects to perform diet collection properly. Moreover, subjects must be reimbursed for the cost of extra food.

When investigating average heavy metal intakes for groups of individuals, it is important to take into consideration the number of days required to obtain a representative number of diet duplicates. One study has shown that even for iron, seven-days diet collections are needed for a group and 68-days for an individual to obtain a true average intake estimate [39]. Although heavy metals were not included in this study, it can be estimated that at least the same number of days

Table 6.4. Estimated average intake of heavy metals (μg/day) from Finnish hospital diets calculated from 11 weekly duplicate diets or by analysis of pooled diet

Heavy metal	Average intake by calculation from analysis of weekly diets	Intake estimated on the basis of analysis of the pooled diet	Difference (%)
Pb	18.6	18.9	1.6
Cd	8.82	9.3	5.2
Hg	1.81	2.0	9.5
Average ± SD			5.4 ± 3.9

or more will be required for heavy metals as for iron. Therefore, in practice, only average intakes of groups may be estimated with this method.

The advantage of the duplicate portion method over the other methods is, however, that data on individual heavy metal intakes and on individual variation in dietary heavy metal intake among populations may be studied. On the other hand, this method is vulnerable to error due to the fact that subjects tend to alter their eating habits during the study period [40].

Relatively few published data are available on heavy metal intakes using the duplicate diet technique [41–44]. More recently, however, this technique seems to have gained more popularity [21,45–49]. Examination of heavy metal intake estimates made for various populations with the duplicate portion method indicates that the estimates are relatively accurate. For example, three heavy metal intake studies in young children in the UK in 1982 [49], 1985 [46] and 1987 [47] yielded very consistent results. Furthermore, the heavy metal intake estimates of retired persons from Sweden made in the 1970s [41,42] are in good agreement with more recent estimates from the same country [50,51].

In Finland, a nationwide hospital diet study was conducted in which 24-h diet duplicates in a seven-day period were collected from all university and central hospitals, then pooled per hospital and homogenized to form 11 one-week diets. An equal percentage of each one-week diet was then sampled, pooled and homogenized to form one mixed average Finnish hospital diet representing 77 individual 24-h diets. The hospital diets were analyzed separately for trace elements including heavy metals and the average value calculated [20,21] compared with the value obtained from analysis of the mixed average hospital diet. The agreement was excellent (Table 6.4) and demonstrates that analytical quality control in the analysis of duplicate diets is relatively easy compared to the analysis of numerous food items of difficult matrices and low concentration levels, as is the case in certain market basket studies.

Comparative Evaluation of the Methods and Conclusions

It is nearly impossible to provide absolute evidence on the validity of the methods discussed here as heavy metal intakes of the same population(s) have never been studied using different methods comparatively at the same time. However, one way of evaluating the validity of heavy metal intake estimates based on dietary analysis is to determine the urinary and fecal heavy metal excretion of the subjects. This method is particularly applicable to cadmium and lead as the average gastrointestinal absorption in adults is known to be approximately 5% [34] and 10% [52], respectively. Naturally, smokers and occupationally exposed persons cannot be included in such evaluations.

Wester [44] found excellent agreement between the ten-day dietary cadmium intake of four Swedish subjects using the duplicate diet method (9.7 µg/day) and their fecal cadmium excretion (8.3 µg/day). By using the duplicate portion techniques, Kjëllström et al. [53] showed that the average fecal excretion of cadmium was 13 µg/day and that of lead was 35 µg/day in Swedish males. The results are in excellent agreement with those reported by Schütz [41] for Swedism males, using the duplicate portion technique, for the average intakes of cadmium (12.9 µg/day) and lead (30 µg/day) at about the same time. More recent studies on cadmium and lead intake in Swedish populations also support the above results [50,51]. As shown previously, lead intake studies conducted in young children in the UK using the duplicate portion technique also yielded very consistent results [43,46,47]. Based on fecal cadmium excretion the average dietary cadmium intake in adults living in US cities has been estimated to be between 12 and 20 µg/day in the early 1970s [34,35]. However, the cadmium intake estimates based on market basket studies from the same period of time were a factor of 2–3 higher in the US [23,27].

It therefore seems justified to conclude that the duplicate portion studies have resulted in more correct estimates for heavy metal intakes, in general, as compared with market basket studies. There are a number of factors affecting the observed discrepancies between the methods. First, inadequate contamination control during sampling, sample handling and analysis which affects more lead than cadmium or mercury intake estimation and studies with high number of samples which is the case with certain market basket studies. Second, inadequate analytical methodology, particularly in terms of sensitivity affects more market basket studies involving a large number of samples with heavy metal contents below the LOQ. Third, duplicate portion studies have become popular only recently as better analytical instrumentation and improved methods of contamination control have been employed.

However, provided that modern analytical instrumentation with minimal sample pretreatment, certified reference materials with similar matrix composition and clean air room facilities for sample handling are used market basket studies also yield correct results as has been shown in Finland [20]. In that study, nine food groups were analyzed separately for heavy metals as well as the entire diet. As shown before, the average intake estimate calculated from the intakes contributed by the food groups was in excellent agreement with the estimate based on the chemical analysis of the entire diet (Table 6.3). Moreover, this average heavy metal intake estimate of the Finns was in excellent agreement with that based on analysis of seven-day hospital diets collected from 11 central hospitals located throughout the country [21] (Table 6.5). The basic composition of the average Finnish hospital

Table 6.5. Average dietary intakes of lead, cadmium and mercury in Finland estimated on the basis of analyses of nationally representative market basket diet compared with those obtained from average hospital duplicate diets

Type of	Lead		Cadmium		Mercury	
	Intake (μg/MJ (ng/kcal))	Intake/PTW[a] (%)	Intake (μg/MJ (ng/kcal))	Intake/PTW[a] (%)	Intake (μg/MJ (ng/kcal))	Intake/PTW[a] (%)
Market basket diet[b]	1.8 (7.5)	4.2	1.0 (4.2)	14.0	0.193 (0.8)	5.3
7-day hospital diet[c]	2.0 (8.3)	4.7	0.96 (4.0)	13.4	0.224 (0.93)	5.9

[a]PTWI = FAO/WHO Provisional Tolerable Weekly Intake [1].
[b]See reference [38].
[c]See reference [21].

diet does not differ markedly from the average Finnish market basket diet, which explains the observed agreement between the estimates.

In conclusion, correct results may be obtained by both methods provided that sophisticated instrumentation as well as dietetic and analytical expertise are available. Then, the focus of the study and prerequisites such as available food consumption data, size of population and the related factors presented above are decisive in the selection of the method to be employed.

References

1. Anonymous (1972) Evaluation of certain food additives and the contaminants: mercury, lead and cadmium. Sixteenth report of the joint FAO/WHO Expert Committee on Food Additives, WHO Technical Report Series no. 505, Geneva
2. Anonymous (1981) Chemical contaminants in food – approaches for estimation of intake. (FAO Food and Nutrition Paper, provisional edition) Food and Agriculture Organization of the United Nations
3. Anonymous (1985) Guidelines for the study of dietary intakes of chemical contaminants. WHO Offset Publication No 87, World Health Organization, Geneva
4. McKenzie HA, Smythe LE (1988) Design of laboratories for trace and ultra-trace analysis. In: McKenzie HA, Smythe LE (eds) Quantitative trace analysis of biological materials. Elsevier, Amsterdam, p 39
5. Horwitz W, Kamps LR, Boyer KW (1980) Quality assurance in the analysis of foods for trace constituents. J Assoc Offic Anal Chem 63:1344–1354
6. Ihnat M (1988) Biological reference materials for quality control. In: McKenzie HA, Smythe LE (eds) Quantitative trace analysis of biological materials. Elsevier, Amsterdam, pp 331–351
7. Dybczyinski R, Veglia A, Suschny O (1980) Report of the intercomparison run A-11 for the determination of inorganic constituents in milk powder. IAEA/RL/68, July 1980. International Atomic Energy Agency, Vienna

8. Parr R (1980) Intercomparison of minor and trace elements in IAEA Animal Muscle (H-4). Report No 2, IAEA/RL/69. International Atomic Energy Agency, Vienna

9. Anonymous (1989) Intercomparison runs/Reference materials 1989. Analytical Quality Control Services. International Atomic Energy Agency, Vienna, Austria

10. Byrne AR, Camara-Rica C, Cornelis R et al. (1987) Results of a co-ordinated research programme to improve the certification of IAEA milk powder A-11 and animal muscle H-4 for eleven "difficult" trace elements. Fresenius Z Anal Chem 326:723–729

11. McKenzie HA (1988) Polarography and stripping voltammetry. In: McKenzie HA, Smythe LE (eds). Quantitative trace analysis of biological materials. Elsevier, Amsterdam, pp 219–240

12. Jones JW (1988) Food samples. In: McKenzie HA, Smythe LE (eds) Quantitative trace analysis of biological materials. Elsevier, Amsterdam, pp 353–365

13. Willis JB, Stevens BJ (1988) Flame emission and atomic absorption spectrometry. In: McKenzie HA, Smythe LE (eds). Quantitative trace analysis of biological materials. Elsevier, Amsterdam, p 135

14. Subramanian KS (1988) Lead. In: McKenzie HA, Smythe LE (eds) Quantitative trace analysis of biological materials. Elsevier, Amsterdam, p. 589

15. Kumpulainen J, Paakki M (1987) Analytical quality control program used by the trace elements in foods and diets sub-network of the FAO European Cooperative method on trace elements. Fresenius Z Anal Chem 326:684–689

16. Kumpulainen J, Paakki M, Tahvonen R (1988) Characterization of a potato reference material for major, minor and trace elements. Fresenius Z Anal Chem 332:685–688

17. Koivistoinen P (ed) (1980) Mineral element composition of Finnish foods: N, K, Mg, P, S, Fe, Cu, Mn, Zn, Mo, Ni, Cr, Se, Si, Rb, Al, B, Br, Hg, As, Cd, Pb and ash. Acta Agric Scand (suppl 22)

18. Louekari K, Salminen S (1986) Intake of heavy metals from foods in Finland, West Germany and Japan. Food Addit Contam 3:355–362

19. Kumpulainen J, Mutanen M, Paakki M, Lehto J (1987) Validity of calculation method in estimating mineral element content of diets. Vån Föda 39 (Suppl 1):75–82

20. Kumpulainen J, Sinisalo M, Paakki M, Tahvonen R (1987) Mineral elements in hospital diets. Kemia-Kemi 14:(Abstract 10.38)

21. Sinisalo M, Kumpulainen J, Paakki M, Tahvonen R (1989) Mineral elements in Finnish hospital diets. In: Chazot G et al. (eds) Current trends in trace elements research. Proceedings of an international symposium, held in Paris, 30–5 November December 1987, Smith-Gordon, London

22. Gunderson EL (1988) FDA total diet study, April 1982–April 1984, dietary intakes of pesticides, selected elements and other chemicals. JAOAC 71:1200–1209

23. Gartrell MJ, Graun JC, Podrebarac DS, Gunderson E (1986) Pesticides selected elements, and other chemicals in adult total diet samples, October 1980–March 1982. JAOAC 69:146–161

24. de Vos RH, van Dokkum W, Olthof PDA, Quirijns JK, Muys T, van der Poll JM (1984) Pesticides and other chemical residues in Dutch total diet samples. Food Chem Toxicol 22:11–21

25. Varo P, Koivistoinen P (1980) General discussion and nutritional evaluation. In: Koivistoninen P (ed) Mineral element comparison of Finnish foods. Acta Agric Scand (Suppl 22), pp 165–171

26. Mutanen M, Kumpulainen J, Lehto J, Koivistoinen P (1985) Comparison of chemical analysis and calculation method in estimating selenium content of Finnish diet. Nutr Res 5:693–697

27. Spickett JT (1979) Cadmium as a food contaminant. Proc Nutr Soc Austr 4:87–94

28. Anonymous (1980) Cadmium Foruening. En vedegotelse om und vendelse, forekomst og skod evirkninger at cadmium in Denmark, Miljöministeriet, Miljöstyrelsen, Strandgade 29, 1401 Copenhagen, Denmark

29. Morgan H, Sherlock JC (1984) Cadmium intake and cadmium in the human kidney. Food Add Contam 1:45–51

30. Anonymous (1977) Report of the 87th session of the National Health and Medical Research Council. Market Basket Survey 1977. Commonwealth of Australia, Canberra, ACT Australian Governement Publishing Service

31. Anonymous (1983) Survey of cadmium in food: first supplementary report. Twelfth Report of the steering group on food surveillance. Ministry of Agriculture, Fisheries and Food, HMSO, London

32. Sillanpää M (1988) Microelements in Finnish soils: study history and current status. Ann Agric Fenn 27:177–190

33. Elias RW (1987) Recent changes in human lead exposure. In: Lindberg SE, Hutchinson TC (eds) International Conference on Heavy Metals in the Environment, New Orleans, 1987, CEP Consultants Ltd, Edinburgh, Page Bros., Norwich, UK, pp 197–202

34. Kowal NE, Johnson DE, Kraemer DF, Pahren HR (1979) Normal levels of cadmium in diet, urine, blood and tissues of inhabitants of the United States. J Toxicol Environ Health 5:995–1014

35. Pahren H, Lucus JB, Ryan JA, Dotson GK (1977) An appraisal of the relative health risks associated with land application of municipal sludge. Paper presented at the fiftieth Annual Conference of the Water Pollution Control Federation, Philadelphia, PA. 2–6 October

36. Yost KJ, Miles CJ, Parsons TW (1980) A method for estimating dietary intake of environmental trace contaminants: Cadmium a case study. Environ Int 3:473–484

37. Kurono T (1983) Lead content in food in Japan in the early 1980's with the estimation of its daily intake. Osaka City Med J 29:15–41

38. Kumpulainen J, Sinisalo M, Paakki M, Tahvonen R (1987) Mineral element content of a nationally representative Finnish market basket diet. Kemia-Kemi 14(Abstract 10B)

39. Basiotis PP, Welse SO, Cronin FJ, Kelsay J, Mertz W (1987) Number of days of food intake records required to estimate individual and group nutrient intakes with defined confidence. J Nutr 117:1638–1641

40. Marr JW Individual dietary surveys: purposes and methods. World Rev Nutr Diet 13:105–109

41. Schütz A (1979) Cadmium and lead. In: Borgström B, Norden Å, Åkesson B, Jägerstad M (eds) Nutrition and old age. Scand J Gastroenterol 14:233–231

42. Schütz A (1979) Mercury. In: Borgstöm B, Norden Å, Åkesson B, Jägerstad M (eds) Nutrition and old age. Scand J Gastroenterol 14:232–235

43. Sherlock J (1982) Assessment of lead intakes and dose–response for a population in Ayr exposed to a plumbosolvent water supply. Human Toxicol 1:115–122

44. Wester PO (1974) Trace element balance in relation to variations in calcium intake. Atherosclerosis 20:207–215

45. Buchet JP, Lauwerys R, Vandevoork A, Pycke JM (1983) Oral daily intake of cadmium, lead, manganese, copper, chromium, mercury, cadmium, zinc, and arsenic in Belgium: a duplicate meal study. Food Chem Toxicol 21:19–24

46. Sherlock JC, Barltrop D, Evans WH, Quirn MJ, Smart GA, Strehlow C (1985) Blood lead concentration and lead intake in children of different ethnic origin. Human Toxicol 4:513–519

47. Smart GA, Sherlock JC, Norman JA (1987) Dietary intakes of lead and other metals: a study of young children from an urban population in the UK. Food Add Contam 5:85–93

48. Dabeka RW, McKenzie AD, Lacroix MA (1987) Dietary intakes of lead, cadmium, arsenic and fluoride by Canadian adults: a 24-h duplicate diet study. Food Add Contam 4:89–102

49. Anonymous (1982) A survey of lead in food: second supplementary report. Tenth report of the steering group on food surveillance. Ministry of Agriculture, Fisheries and Food, HMSO, London

50. Slorach S, Gustafsson J-B, Jorhem L, Mattsson P (1983) Intake of lead, cadmium and certain other metals via a typical Swedish weekly diet. Vår Föda 35:1–16 (Suppl 1/83)

51. Becker W, Kumpulainen J (1991) Contents of essential and toxic mineral elements in Swedish market basket diet in 1987. Br J Nutr (In press)

52. Anonymous (1977) Environmental health criteria 3 – Lead. World Health Organization, Geneva

53. Kjellström T, Borg K, Lind B (1978) Cadmium in feces as an estimate of daily cadmium intake in Sweden. Environ Res 15:242–251

CHAPTER 7

Risks of Dietary Exposure to Pesticides in Infants and Children

D. Krewski,[1] J. Wargo,[2] and R. Rizek[3]

Introduction

Each year in the United States, approximately 2.7 billion pounds of insecticides, fungicides, herbicides, rodenticides, nematicides, and other chemicals are used to control a variety of living organisms collectively named "pests" [1]. Nearly 600 active chemical ingredients are combined with 1200 inert ingredients in various formulations to produce approximately 50 000 different pesticide products.

The US Environmental Protection Agency (EPA) is responsible for setting tolerances for pesticide residues in foods. There are nearly 8500 pesticide-crop residue tolerances listed within the US Code of Federal Regulations [2] representing maximum residues of 300 active chemical ingredients permitted by EPA to exist in food. For example, 100 different chemicals have approved tolerances for tomatoes, 88 for potatoes, 112 for apples, and 108 for corn.

At the request of the US Congress, and with the support of the US Environmental Protection Agency, the US National Research Council initiated a study in 1988 to examine risk assessment methods for pesticides in the diet, focusing on infants and children. To conduct the study, the National Research Council created the Committee on Pesticides in the Diets of Infants and Children. This Committee is established jointly under the Commission on Life Sciences, Board on Environmental Studies and Toxicology, and the Board on Agriculture.

The study will evaluate current risk assessment methods in light of the potential sensitivities and increased exposure of infants and children. This study derives from the general consensus in the scientific community that new methods may be available to improve risk assessment methods and thus better protect the public health. It is important to note, however, that this study does not

[1]Health Protection Branch, Health and Welfare Canada, Ottawa, Ontario. Canada K1A 0L2.
[2]School of Forestry and Environmental Studies, Yale University, New Haven, Connecticut 06511, USA.
[3]Human Nutrition Information Service, US Department of Agriculture, Hyattsville, Maryland 20782, USA.

arise from any documented increase in adverse health conditions in infant, children, or adults resulting from exposure to pesticides in the diet.

The purpose of this chapter is to discuss data sources and methodological issues relevant to this study. General survey methods for determining food consumption levels are considered, followed by actual food monitoring surveys that have been conducted in the United States. Some preliminary data on food consumption patterns for infants and children in relation to the US population as a whole are presented. The determination of dietary intakes of pesticides using information on pesticide residues in food is discussed briefly and approaches to health risk assessment are outlined with special reference to infants and children.

Methods for Determining Dietary Intakes

Several different approaches are available for determining food consumption patterns [3]. Retrospective methods require individuals to recall foods eaten in the past. These methods include 24-hour food recalls and food frequency questionnaires. Prospective methods require individuals to keep a record or diary of foods and beverages consumed as eaten. A combination of retrospective and prospective methods can be used to improve the accuracy of the dietary information obtained [4].

24-Hour Dietary Recall

With the 24-hour recall method, individuals are asked to list and describe from memory all foods consumed during the past 24 hours. This approach has been used in large-scale dietary surveys [5,6] and in large-scale studies of diet and health [7,8]. In panel studies [9] several 24-hour recalls have been obtained during the course of a year.

The strengths of the 24-hour recall include fast and easy administration, thereby minimizing respondent burden. The short time period for recall avoids telescoping bias, and normal food habits are unchanged by the reporting procedure. Limitations of the method include reliance on the respondent's memory, and the need to probe for omission of food items. Although the method can provide reliable estimates of the mean intake for large population groups, one 24-hour recall is unlikely to be representative of an individual's usual intake. However, individual information can be improved upon using multiple recalls done on different days.

Food Frequency Questionnaire

In its simplest form, the food frequency questionnaire consists of a checklist of foods or food groups and a set of response categories indicating how often each food was consumed during a specified time period, often a few weeks, few months, or a year [10]. The list of foods may be short (under 20 items) or long (over 100 items), so that completion of the questionnaire (either interviewer or self-administered) may take from 10 minutes to more than one hour.

This approach to determining food consumption patterns has been validated to some extent by comparison with actual records of food intake [11–13]. It provides a relatively simple low-cost method of obtaining information on long-term individual food consumption patterns, including individuals whose intakes of certain foods are notably above average. The method does rely on accurate recall over a relatively long time period, and may thus be inappropriate for children. Particular food frequency questionnaires may be inappropriate for individuals who have unusual diets or consume foods not included in the questionnaire list.

Food Diary

The food record or food diary is a written or spoken report of current food intake, usually for a short but defined period of time ranging from 1 day to 4 weeks. Longer periods of up to one year have been reported in some studies [14]. Subjects are asked to list all foods and beverages ingested and to record descriptions and portion amounts immediately after consumption. Portions may be weighed or measured before eating when at home. The food record is usually self-administered, although children and others unable to report for themselves may require a knowledgeable surrogate to do the recording. The food record approach to consumption monitoring is generally considered to be more accurate than recall methods [15] and has been widely used as the standard for validation of other methods.

The food diary method places little reliance on memory, and minimizes the potential for omission of foods and beverages that have been consumed. Its greatest weakness is the heavy recording burden placed on respondents, who must be literate and co-operative to ensure success. In addition, food obtained and eaten away from home may be less well described and quantified than food prepared at home. Accuracy of reporting may also decline if the time period is lengthy because of respondent boredom or fatigue.

Food Consumption Surveys

Early studies on food and nutrition were conducted at the end of the last century. These were small-scale studies aimed at helping people achieve good diets at low cost. In the United States, the first survey of national scope was a supplement to the Consumer Purchases Study of 1935–37, conducted jointly by several federal agencies. Since then, the US Department of Agriculture has conducted six major (decennial) national food consumption surveys. Until 1965, the surveys were limited to the collection of information on the quantities of foods used by households and the cost of those foods. In the 1965–66 survey, the homemaker was asked to recall the dietary intakes of certain household members for the day prior to the interview.

Nationwide Food Consumption Survey (1977–78)

In the 1977–78 Nationwide Food Consumption Survey (NFCS), dietary intakes for three consecutive days were collected in four seasons from specified individuals in sample households. The data were collected using a 1-day recall and a 2-day food diary. The three days of dietary intake data provided a better measure of an individual's average intake than did the 1-day measure used in 1965.

Continuing Survey of Food Intakes (1985–86)

In 1985, the US Department of Agriculture initiated the Continuing Survey of Food Intakes by Individuals. This survey was repeated in 1986. Beginning in 1989 it will be conducted on an annual basis. This series of surveys was initiated to respond to a generally perceived need for ongoing data on the adequacy of diets of the general population and subpopulations at high nutritional risk.

The 1985 and 1986 surveys included the collection of six non-consecutive days of intake using a 1-day recall for each day of dietary data. In both 1985 and 1986, the information was collected bimonthly to provide six 1-day food recalls for each household member completing the survey. The purpose of collecting six non-consecutive days of intake was to provide a better measure of usual intake. However, collecting non-consecutive days of data was costly and response rates over the full year were not as high as expected. Therefore, future surveys will include the collection of three consecutive days of intake information (1-day recall and 2 day record) as in the National Food Consumption Survey of 1977–78.

In the 1985 and 1986 surveys, data were collected from approximately 1500 women and 500 of their children. Only women aged 19 to 50 years and their children ages 1 through 5, if any, were designated for sample selection. These groups were chosen because previous surveys have shown that they are more likely than other population groups to have diets low in some nutrients.

National Food Consumption Survey (1987–88)

In 1987–88, the Department of Agriculture returned to the method used in 1977–78, that is, the collection of three consecutive days of intake information based on a combination 1-day recall and 2-day diary. This change was due, in part, to response rate problems with the six non-consecutive days and in part to funding limitations. As in 1977–78, individual food intake interviews in 1987–88 followed completion of the household food use interview with the person primarily responsible for planning and preparing meals. Also, the 1987–88 National Food Consumption Survey included all individuals ratheɬ than the limited sex/age groups of the Continuing Surveys of Food Intakes by Individuals conducted in 1985 and 1986.

In the 1987–88 National Food Consumption Survey, all members of the household were eligible to be interviewed individually if they were 12 years or older and were able to report for themselves. The 1-day recall was interviewer-administered and interviewer-recorded. Interviewers used a set of measuring cups, spoons, and ruler to help respondents estimate portions consumed. After completing the recall, the interviewer instructed respondents in keeping the 2-day record. Interviewers later returned to review and pick up completed records. Monetary incentives were paid for completing each 3-day report: $2.00 per individual 3-day report up to a maximum of $20.00 per household. Monetary incentives were paid in 1977–78 but not in 1985–86.

Food Consumption Patterns

The surveys discussed in the previous section may be used to develop food consumption profiles for infants and children. The results presented here are based upon the 1977–78 US Department of Agriculture food consumption survey of 30 770 individuals. Although this survey is subject to certain limitations (including its age, the fact that it was conducted only over one three-day period, and the small sample size of nursing infants), it does represent the most comprehensive database currently available to compare all age classes within the population at large. For present purposes, the most important limitation is that the survey reflects consumption patterns at a single point in time, whereas it is likely that dietary patterns change quickly in response to changing tastes, marketing strategies, advances in food processing technology, and medical restrictions.

Individual consumption reports were broken into 376 different types of foods and 691 forms of those foods. To facilitate data analysis, Wargo [16] has created a microcomputer-based database which breaks down the consumption data by year and other demographic variables. Average consumption was calculated for the 376 different types of food, and for 22 different age classes which have been aggregated into five major classes including non-nursing infants between the age of birth and 1 year, children aged 1–6 years, children 7–12 years, teenagers, and adults over 20 years.

These data were used to identify all foods representing at least 1% (by weight) of the average US diet. For each age class, the average intake of each of these foods relative to the US average could then be determined (Table 7.1). In general, infants and children consumed proportionately more of these foods than did the population at large.

Twenty-two foods constitute more than 1% of the average non-nursing infant's diet, the top 15 of which are listed in Table 7.2. Six of these are fruits, which together account for 29% of the diet. Nine fruits or vegetables comprise 37% of the diet. Soy and coconut oil together account for approximately 5% of the diet, most likely from infant formulae. Non-nursing infant consumption of soy oil is 4.6 times higher than the US average level, whereas coconut oil consumption is 50 times the US average, a fact which could have significant implications for the regulation of fat-soluble pesticides. Milk products constitute over 21% of the average non-nursing infant's diet, 7.3 times the US average for non-fat milk solids intake and 3.6 times the US average for fat milk solids. These data indicate the

Table 7.1. Foods representing at least 1% (by weight) of the average US diet and age class consuming highest multiple above US average consumption

Commodity	% of diet	Age class consuming highest multiple	Multiple of US average consumption level
1. Wheat flour	7.4	Children 1–6	2.25
2. Lean beef	6.9	Children 1–6	1.82
3. Orange juice	6.7	Children 1–6	3.08
4. Non-fat milk	5.4	Non-nursing infants	7.33
5. Pulp potato	4.7	Children 1–6	2.14
6. Cane sugar	4.4	Children 1–6	2.49
7. Whole eggs	3.3	Children 1–6	2.30
8. Whole tomatoes	2.9	Children 1–6	1.68
9. Fresh apples	2.8	Non-nursing infants	6.91
10. Milk-fat solids	2.5	Non-nursing infants	3.62
11. Lean pork	2.3	Children 1–6	1.84
12. Chicken (incl. skin)	2.3	Children 1–6	2.15
13. Beef-fat	2.2	Children 1–6	1.81
14. Whole potatoes	2.1	Children 1–6	1.79
15. Beet sugar	1.9	Children 1–6	2.49
16. Soybean oil	1.9	Non-nursing infants	4.55
17. Apple juice	1.4	Non-nursing infants	16.65
18. Sweet corn	1.4	Children 1–6	2.39
19. Fresh bananas	1.4	Non-nursing infants	4.96
20. Fresh peaches	1.3	Non-nursing infants	10.60
21. Head of lettuce	1.3	Nursing mothers	1.57
22. Pork fat	1.2	Children 1–6	2.10
23. Green beans	1.2	Non-nursing infants	4.65
24. Salted finned fish	1.1	Nursing mothers	2.41
25. Garden peas	1.0	Non-nursing infants	3.72
26. Carrots	1.0	Non-nursing infants	9.05
27. Pureed tomatoes	1.0	Children 1–6	2.15
28. Corn	1.0	Hispanics	3.37
29. Milled rice	1.0	Non-nursing infants	8.69

importance of monitoring both the percentage of total diet and the multiple of the US average consumption level as critical indicators of concern for estimating dietary exposure to pesticides.

Adult food consumptions differ notably from those of small children (Table 7.3). Beef represents the most consumed food, while intake of wheat flour, orange juice, potatoes and milk decline slightly from teenage levels. The list of the 15 most consumed foods is almost identical for both teenagers and adults, and diversity of foods increases again with age, although this may be the result of the large adult sample size. Similarly, adult food intake is close to the US average.

Table 7.2. Fifteen most consumed foods by non-nursing infants

Food	% of diet (by weight)	Multiple of US average
1. Non-fat milk solids	12.3	7.3
2. Apple juice	7.5	16.7
3. Milk sugar (lactose)	6.3	79.1
4. Fresh apples	6.0	6.9
5. Orange juice	5.9	2.9
6. Fresh peaches	4.4	10.6
7. Fresh pears	3.6	15.0
8. Carrots	2.9	9.1
9. Milk-fat solids	2.9	3.6
10. Lean beef	2.8	1.3
11. Soybean oil	2.7	4.6
12. Milled rice	2.7	8.7
13. Coconut oil	2.5	49.8
14. Fresh bananas	2.1	5.0
15. Wheat flour	1.8	0.8

Differences in dietary patterns between 1977–78 and 1985–86–87 are currently being analyzed; however, several trends appear to be emerging. First, and perhaps most important, there appears to be a fair degree of consistency in dietary patterns among young children over time. For example, the same foods appear among the top 10 most consumed by children aged 1–5 years for both

Table 7.3. Fifteen most consumed foods by adults (20 years and older)

Food	% of diet (by weight)	Multiple of US average intake
1. Lean beef	7.6	0.83
2. Wheat flour	7.0	0.71
3. Orange juice	5.5	0.61
4. Potato pulp	4.7	0.74
5. Cane sugar	3.7	0.64
6. Whole eggs	3.7	0.83
7. Whole tomatoes	3.4	0.88
8. Milk non-fat solids	3.3	0.47
9. Lean pork	2.7	0.87
10. Whole potatoes	2.5	0.90
11. Beef – fat	2.4	0.83
12. Chicken (including skin)	2.4	0.79
13. Fresh apples	2.1	0.58
14. Milk fat solids	1.9	0.57
15. Soybean oil	1.9	0.75

survey periods. Second, in the latest survey, fruits and fruit juices constitute a larger percentage of the average diet during the first few years of life than they did a decade ago. Third, dietary diversity increases with age in both survey periods. Fourth, consumption patterns of teenagers appear to approach US average levels. Fifth, small children consume several times the adult average intake of the most consumed foods when adjusted for body weight.

Dietary Intake of Pesticides

Determination of dietary intake of pesticides requires information on residue levels in foods in addition to food consumption data. A theoretical daily intake level can be obtained by assuming that pesticides are present in all foods on which their use is permitted at the established tolerance [17]. This theoretical daily intake can overestimate actual intake since not all foods are treated with pesticides registered for use on the corresponding crop. Residue levels can also be affected by the method of food preparation. For example, boiling certain vegetables can volatilize water-soluble chemical residues, and hence reduce exposure. In practice, market basket surveys conducted by the Food and Drug Administration [18] suggest that residues on raw commodities are frequently well below the tolerance level [19,20].

A more accurate approach to exposure estimation is direct measurement of pesticide residues in a more complete selection of foods than is included in market basket studies. Unfortunately, comprehensive nationwide residue monitoring studies are prohibitively expensive, and have not been implemented. Nonetheless, residue data collected from surveillance of selected food products will be of some use in gauging the extent to which the theoretical daily intake may reflect actual intake [21,22].

Risk Assessment

Toxicological Risk Assessment

The regulation of toxicants without the capacity to induce carcinogenic or mutagenic effects has traditionally been based on the concept that there is a level of exposure below which a health effect is not expected, even if exposure occurs over a lifetime. The existence of a so-called "threshold" dose is supported by the observation that the toxicity of many agents is manifest only after the depletion of a known physiological reserve, and that the biological repair capacity of many organisms can accommodate a certain degree of damage by reversible toxic processes [23,24]. Above this threshold, however, the homeostatic physiological processes which allow compensatory mechanisms to maintain normal biological function may be overwhelmed, leading to organ dysfunction. The objective of classical toxicological risk assessment is thus to establish a threshold dose below which adverse health effects are not expected to occur.

Historically, this concept was first introduced by Lehman and Fitzhugh [25], who proposed that an acceptable daily intake (ADI) could be calculated for contaminants in human food. Formally, the acceptable daily intake was defined by

$$ADI = NOAEL/SF$$

where the NOAEL is the no-observed adverse effect level in toxicological studies, and the safety factor (SF) is selected to allow for differences in sensitivity to the test agent in humans as compared to animals, and for variation in sensitivity within the human population. These two sources of variation were often accommodated through the use of a $10 \times 10 = 100$-fold safety factor [26].

In 1977, the US National Research Council Safe Drinking Water Committee reviewed the methods that had evolved for establishing ADIs, and made several significant recommendations. First, the Committee proposed that the NOAEL be expressed in mg/kg body weight rather than mg/kg diet to adjust for differences in dietary consumption patterns. Second, the Committee explicitly supported the use of only a 10-fold safety factor in the presence of dose–response data derived from human studies. And third, the Committee proposed an additional 10-fold safety factor in the absence of adequate toxicity data, for an overall safety factor of 1000-fold. In summary, the essential recommendations of the Safe Drinking Water Committee can be expressed as follows [27].

SF = 10: Based on human studies involving prolonged ingestion, with no indication of carcinogenicity.

SF = 100: Based on results of chronic toxicity studies in one or more species, with no indication of carcinogenicity. Human data are either unavailable or scanty.

SF = 1000: Based on acute or subchronic toxicity data, with no indication of carcinogenicity. Neither chronic toxicity or acute human are available.

Although the use of safety factors is now accepted practice in toxicological risk assessment, the limitations of these approaches should also be emphasized. Since the ADI is only an estimate of the population threshold or true no-effect level, it does not provide absolute assurance of safety. The size of the safety factor is not directly related to sample size, so that smaller experiments would tend to lead to large ADIs than would larger more sensitive studies. Although factors of 10-fold are used to accommodate both inter- and intra-species variation in sensitivity, it cannot be guaranteed that a 100-fold safety factor will afford adequate protection in this regard in all cases. For these reasons, the ADI should not be viewed as possessing a high degree of mathematical precision, but rather as a guide to human exposure levels which are not expected to present serious health risks.

Recently, the US Environmental Protection Agency has recommended using the term "uncertainty factor" (UF) rather than "safety factor" in recognition that the ADI does not guarantee absolute safety and has relabeled the ADI as a reference dose or RfD [28]. The agency also introduced the concept of a modifying factor (MF) to be applied to the UF in recognition of the specific circumstances surrounding the establishment of the RfD. The calculated ADI for specific chemicals allowed the assumption that food containing the chemical could be safely consumed daily by humans, including sensitive subgroups, for a lifetime without inducing harmful effects. Thus, the RfD is determined by use of the equation

$$RfD = NAOEL/(UF \times MF)$$

where the NOAEL is the highest dose at which there is no statistically significant adverse effect in the test animals beyond that exhibited by a control group, UF is an uncertainty factor which accommodates uncertainties in the extrapolation of dose-threshold data to humans, and MF is a modifying factor sometimes invoked when scientific uncertainties in the study are not accommodated by the uncertainty factor. When the data do not demonstrate a NOAEL, a LOAEL (lowest-observed-adverse-effect level) may be used.

Carcinogen Risk Assessment

The regulation of carcinogens is considered a unique issue in risk assessment due to the lack of evidence of a threshold dose. The absence of such a threshold implies that any non-zero level of exposure may confer some risk. To evaluate the significance of low levels of exposure, it is often useful to estimate the potential risk associated with such exposures.

The quantitative description of neoplastic processes requires a mathematical model of carcinogenesis. The multistage model has a long history of use in theoretical descriptions of carcinogenesis [29]. The multistage model is based on the promise that a stem cell must sustain a series of mutations in order to give rise to a malignant cancer cell, and provides a good description of many forms of human cancer by allowing for between two and six stages. Moolgavkar et al. [30,31] have proposed a two-stage model which provides an equally good fit to these same data by explicitly allowing for tissue growth and cell kinetics. This biologically motivated model of carcinogenesis based on the hypothesis that a tumor may be initiated following the occurrence of genetic damage in one or more cells in the target tissue as a result of exposure to an initiator. Such initiated cells may then undergo malignant transformation to give rise to a cancerous lesion. The rate of occurrence of such lesions may be increased by subsequent exposure to a promoter, which serves to increase the pool of initiated cells through mechanisms that result in clonal expansion.

In the absence of epidemiological data, carcinogenic risk assessment is necessarily based on laboratory studies using animal models for humans [32]. Because such tests are generally conducted at high doses to elicit measurable response rates in relatively small experimental groups, low dose risk assessment is generallly done by downward extrapolation of results obtained at higher doses. Although the choice of the dose–response model to be used for extrapolation purposes can have a marked impact on estimates of low dose risk [33], such differences are small when attention is restricted to models which are linear in the low dose region. The assumption of low dose linearity for chemical carcinogens which act through direct interaction with genetic material is supported by both theoretical considerations in carcinogenesis [34] and the linearity of DNA binding observed at very low doses with a number of chemical carcinogens [35]. Although perhaps not applicable in certain cases, such as when carcinogenesis only occurs subsequent to toxic tissue injury, the assumption of low dose linearity is widely made in regulatory applications of low dose risk assessment in the absence of clear information to the contrary [36].

As a practical matter, the US Environmental Protection Agency [37] uses the linearized multistage model (LMS) to obtain estimates of low dose risk. This is done by obtaining an upper confidence limit q_i^* on the linear component of the model [38]. The value of q_i^* represents the slope of the dose–response curve in the low dose region, and is equal to the risk associated with a unit measure of dose (such as 1 mg/kg/day). Only an upper confidence limit on this low dose slope is used on the grounds that the maximum likelihood estimate of this parameter is highly unstable. Other approaches to linear extrapolation have also been proposed [39], although these generally lead to risk estimates close to those provided by the LMS.

For purposes of human risk assessment, animal cancer potency values need to be converted to humans. Qualitatively, this presumes that positive animal cancer tests are predictive of similar effects in humans [32]. Quantitatively, potency values may be converted on a body weight surface area basis [40], although empirical studies of the correlation between animal and human cancer potency values provide little basis for choosing between these two methods of species conversion [41]. Recent re-analyses of existing data on antineoplastic agents suggest that an intermediate scaling factor based on body weight to the 3/4 power may be most appropriate [42].

The US Environmental Protection Agency has developed a "List of Oncogenic Compounds and Suspects" which summarizes the oncogenic classification of chemical carcinogens and their potency q_i^*. The list includes 99 chemicals, several of which have been cancelled for food use by the EPA. The Agency has developed oncogenic potency factors in human equivalents for 61 of these chemicals, based on a surface area approach to species conversion. These values have been used by the National Research Council [43] and the National Resources Defense Council [44] in assessing the potential risks of dietary exposure to pesticides.

Risk Assessment for Infants and Children

Traditional risk assessment methods generally do not make specific allowances for any unique features of infants and children [45]. Species conversion of dietary intakes done on a body weight basis are normally based on adult body weight and food consumption data [46]. Babich and Davis [47] note that children may be hypersusceptible to food toxicants, particularly heavy metals and pesticides. Gaines and Linder [48] recently estimated the LD_{50}s for 28 pesticides in adult and weanling rats, and found four cases (promotion, atrazine, ametryne and simazine) in which the weanlings were more sensitive than the adult. The process of atherosclerosis is now known to begin in childhood, and has led to recommendations to reduce the total fat intake of children to 30% of calories in children over two years of age, and to limit cholesterol intake to a maximum of 300 mg daily [49].

In assessing the potential carcinogenic risks faced by infants and children, consideration needs to be given to unique physiological sensitivities as well as the age at which exposure occurs. In a study of the carcinogenic effects of *n*-nitroso compounds in the diets of rats conducted by the British Industrial Biological Research Association, for example, a sixfold difference in liver tumor rates were observed between animals exposed for the balance of their lifetimes beginning at 3 and 20 weeks of age [50]. Other studies have identified perinatal exposure as a critical factor in neoplastic development. During the 1970s three independent two-generation cancer bioassays involving *in utero* exposure produced a highly significant increase in the incidence of malignant tumors in the urinary bladders of male rats, whereas no such effects were observed in single generation studies [51]. Although these results suggested that in utero exposure is necessary for bladder tumor induction, a subsequent study conducted by the International Research and Development Corporation (IRDC) produced tumor yields comparable to those observed in the two-generation studies in animals exposed only from birth onwards [52]. The critical difference between the IRDC study and previous single generation studies was the commencement of exposure at birth rather than the time of weaning.

Recently, both the multistage model and the two-stage clonal expansion models have been extended so as to accommodate the age at which exposure occurs [53–55]. These results indicate that when an early stage in the carcinogenic process is dose dependent, early exposures will be of greater concern than later exposures. In this case, equivalent exposures will present greater risks to infants and children than to adults. The extent to which infants and children will be at greater risk depends on the particular assumptions made concerning the mechanism of carcinogenesis. In the classical multistage model this increase may be limited to a multiplicative factor equal to the number of stages included in the model. With the two-stage clonal expansion model, however, the increased risk can be substantial when the agent of interest greatly increases the proliferation rate of the initiated cell population.

Conclusions

This chapter has discussed a number of issues involved in the assessment of potential health risks associated with dietary exposure to pesticides. Based on this discussion, it is clear that an evaluation of risks to infants and children will be particularly difficult. Nonetheless, the Committee on Pesticides in the Diets of Infants and Children plans to review critically food consumption survey methods, pesticide residue detection methods and sampling procedures, and available information on the actual levels of pesticides to which infants and children are exposed. The usefulness of animal testing and extrapolation models, sensitivities of children to toxic substances, and the ultimate effect of these factors on methods used to project lifetime risk will also be examined. Ultimately, the Committee will seek improvements in the risk assessment process that will better protect infants and children from potential health effects from exposures to pesticides in the diet, that may occur either in childhood or later in life.

References

1. US Environmental Protection Agency (1988) Pesticide industry sales and usage: 1987 market estimates. Office of Pesticide Programs, Environmental Protection Agency, Washington, DC
2. US Code of Federal Regulations (1989) Title 21, Part 193; Title 40, Part 180. US Government Printing Office, Washington, DC
3. Dwyer JT (1988) Assessment of dietary intake. In: Shuls ME, Young VR (eds). Modern Nutrition in Health and Disease, 7th edn, Lea & Febiger, Philadelphia, pp 887–905
4. National Research Council (1989) Diet and Health: Implications for Reducing Chronic Disease Risk. National Academy Press, Washington, DC
5. US Department of Agriculture (1972) Food and nutrient intake of individuals in the United States, spring 1965. Household Food Consumption Survey 1965–66, Rep. No. 11, US Department of Agriculture, Hyattsville, Maryland
6. US Department of Health and Human Services (1983) Dietary intake source data: United States, 1976–80. DHHS Pub. No. (PHS) 83-1681, Superintendent of Documents, Washington, DC
7. Tillotson JL, Gorder DD, Kassim N (1981) Nutrition data collection in the multiple risk factor intervention trial. J Am Diet Assoc 78:235–240
8. Frank GC, Voors AW, Schilling PE, Berenson GS (1977) Dietary studies of rural school children in a cardiovascular survey. J Am Diet Assoc 71:31–35
9. US Department of Agriculture (1987) Continuing survey of food intakes by individuals: women 19–50 years and their children 1–5 years, 4 days, 1985. NFCS, CSFII Rep. No. 85-4, US Department of Agriculture, Hyattsville, Maryland
10. Sampson L (1985) Food frequency questionnaire as a research instrument. Clin Nutr 4:171–178
11. Freudenheim JL, Johnson NE, Wardrop RL (1987) Misclassification of nutrient intake of individuals and groups using one-, two-, three-, and seven-day food records. Am J Epidemiol 126:703–713
12. Willett WC, Sampson L, Stampfer MJ, et al. (1985) Reproducibility and validity of a semiquantified food frequency questionnaire. Am J Epidemiol 122:51–65
13. Chu SY, Kolonel LN, Hankin JH, Lee J (1984) A comparison of frequency and quantitative dietary methods for epidemiologic studies of diet and disease. Am J Epidemiol 119:323–334
14. Basiotis PP, Welsh SO, Cronin FJ, Kensay JL, Mertz W (1987) Number of days of food intake records required to estimate individual and group nutrient intakes with defined confidence. J Nutr 117:1638–1641
15. Marr JW, Heady JA (1986) Within- and between-person variation in dietary surveys: number of days needed to classify individuals. Hum Nutr Appl Nutr 40A:347–364

16. Wargo J (1987) Analytical methodology for estimating oncongenic risks for human exposure to agricultural chemicals in food crops. In: Regulating pesticides in food: the Delaney paradox. National Academy Press, Washington, DC, pp 174–195

17. Schmidt RD (1989) Guidelines for predicting dietary intakes of pesticide residues. Prepared with the Joint UNEP/FAO/WHO Food Contamination Monitoring Program in collaboration with the Codex Committee on Pesticide Residues. World Health Organization, Geneva

18. Gunderson EL (1988) FDA total diet study, April. 1982–April 1984, dietary intakes of pesticides, selected elements, and other chemicals. J Assoc Off Anal Chem 71:1200–1209

19. US Food and Drug Administration (1988) Food and Drug Administration pesticide program: residues in foods–1987. J Assoc Off Anal Chem 71:156A–174A

20. Archibald SO, Winter CK (1989) Pesticide residues and cancer risks. Calif Agric 43:6–9

21. Office of Technology Assessment (1988) Pesticide Residues in Food: technologies for detection. US Government Printing Office, Washington, DC

22. Fan AM, Jackson RJ (1989) Pesticides and food safety. Regul Toxicol Pharmacol 9:158–174

23. Klaasen CD (1986) Principles of toxicology. In: Klaasen CD, Amdur MO, Doull J (eds) Macmillan, New York, pp 11–32

24. Aldridge WN (1986) The biological basis and measurement of thresholds. Ann Rev Pharmacol Toxicol 26:39–58

25. Lehman AJ, Fitzhugh OG (1954) 100-fold margin of safety. Assoc Food Drug Off USO Bull 18:33–35

26. National Research Council (1970) Evaluating the safety of food chemicals. National Academy Press, Washington, DC

27. National Research Council (1977) Drinking water and health. National Academy Press, Washington, DC

28. Barnes DG, Dourson ML (1988) Reference dose (RfD): description and use in health assessments. Reg Toxicol Pharmacol 8:471–486

29. Armitage P (1985) Multistage models of carcinogenesis. Environ Health Perpsect 63:195–201

30. Moolgavkar SH (1986) Carcinogenesis modeling from molecular biology to epidemiology. Ann Rev Public Health 7:151–169

31. Moolgavkar SH (1986) Hormones and multistage carcinogenesis. Cancer Surveys 5:635–648

32. Rall DP, Hogan MD, Huff JE, Schwetz BA, Tenant RW (1987) Alternatives to using human experience in assessing health risks. Ann Rev Public Health 8:355–385

33. Krewski D, Van Ryzin J (1981) Dose response models for quantal response toxicity data. In: Csorgo M, Dawson D, Rao JNK, Saleh E (eds) Statistics and related topics. North Holland, Amsterdam, pp 201–231

34. Krewski D, Murdoch D, Withey J (1989) Recent developments in carcinogenic risk assessment. Health Phys 57(Suppl 1):313–325

35. Lutz WK, Buss P, Baertsch A, Caviezel M (1990) Evaluation of DNA binding in vivo for low dose extrapolation in chemical carcinogenesis. In: Waters MD, Nesnow S, Lewtas J, Moore NM, Daniel FB (eds) Genetic toxicology of complex mixtures. Plenum, New York. In press.

36. Office of Science and Technology Policy (1985) Chemical carcinogens: a review of the science and its associated principles. Federal Register 50:10372–10442

37. US Environmental Protection Agency (1986) Guidelines for carcinogen risk assessment. Federal Register 51:33992–34003
38. Crump KS (1984) An improved procedure for low-dose carcinogenic risk assessment from minimal data. J Environ Pathol Toxicol Oncol 6:339–348
39. Krewski D, Gaylor DW, Szyszkowicz MS (1990) A model-free approach to low dose extrapolation. Environ Health Perspectives.
40. Krewski D, Goddard MJ, Withey J (1990) Carcinogenic potency and interspecies extrapolation. In: Mendelsohn ML (ed) Proceedings of the Fifth International Conference in Environmental Mutagents. Alan R Liss, New York.
41. Allen B, Crump KS, Shipp A (1988) Carcinogenic potency of chemicals in animals and humans. Risk Anal 8:531–544
42. Travis CC, Whyte RK (1988) Interspecific scaling of toxicity data. Risk Anal 8:119–125
43. National Research Council (1987) Regulating pesticides in foods: the Delaney paradox. National Academy Press, Washington, DC
44. Natural Resources Defence Council (1989) Intolerable risk: pesticides in our children's food. Natural Resources Defence Council, New York
45. International Program on Chemical Safety (1986) Principles for evaluating health risks from chemicals during infancy and early childhood: The need for a special approach. Environmental Health Criteria 59, World Health Organization, Geneva
46. McColl S (1989) Biological safety factors in toxicological risk assessment. Health and Welfare Canada, Ottawa
47. Babich H, Davis DL (1981) Food tolerances and action levels: do they adequately protect children? BioScience 31:429–438
48. Gaines TB, Linder RE (1989) Acute toxicity of pesticides in adult and weanling rats. Fundam Appl Toxicol 7:299–308
49. American Health Foundation (1989) Coronary artery disease prevention: cholesterol – a pediatric perspective. Prev Med 18:323–409
50. Peto R, Gray R, Brantom P, Grasso P (1986) Nitrosamine carcinogenesis in 5120 rodents: chronic administration of sixteen different concentrations of NDEA, NDMA, NPYR and NPIP in the water of 4440 inbred rats, with parallel studies on NDEA alone of the effect of age of starting (3, 6 or 20 weeks) and of species (rats, mice or hamsters). In: L'Neil IK, Von Borstel RC, Miller CT, Long J, Bartsch H (eds) N-Nitroso compounds: occurrence, biological effects and relevance to human cancer. IARC Scientific Publications No. 57, IARC, Lyon, pp 627–665
51. Arnold DL, Krewski D, Munro IC (1983) Saccharin: a toxicological and historical perspective. Toxicology 27:179–256
52. Anonymous (1985) Saccharin: current status. Food Chem Toxicol 23:417–546
53. Kodell RL, Gaylor DW, Chen JJ (1987) Using average lifetime dose rate for intermitten exposures to carcinogens. Risk Anal 7:339–345
54. Chen JJ, Kodell RL, Gaylor D (1988) Using the biological two-stage model to assess risk from short-term exposures. Risk Anal 8:223–230
55. Murdoch D, Krewski D (1988) Carcinogenic risk assessment with time-dependent exposure patterns. Risk Anal 8:521–530

CHAPTER 8

Use of Intake Data in Risk Assessments by JECFA/JMPR and in Codex Decisions

J.L. Herrman[1]

The Joint FAO/WHO Expert Committee on Food Additives (JECFA) and the Joint FAO/WHO Meeting on Pesticide Residues (JMPR) have both been meeting regularly for many years. Since the mid-1950s, when the first JECFA meeting was held [1], the Committee has evaluated more than 700 different substances, primarily food additives, but also contaminants and, recently, veterinary drugs. JMPR first met in 1963 [2], and since then approximately 200 pesticides have been evaluated.

Since JECFA and JMPR are joint committees, Secretariats in both the Food and Agriculture Organization of the United Nations and in the World Health Organization are responsible for organizing and running them. The WHO Secretariat has been the responsibility of the International Programme on Chemical Safety (IPCS) since the time of its inception in 1980. IPCS is a joint venture of the United Nations Environment Programme, the International Labour Organisation, and the World Health Organization, the main objective of which is to carry out and disseminate evaluations of the effects of chemicals on human health and the environment. It is likely that FAO will soon be joining IPCS as one of the co-operating institutions.

Both JECFA and JMPR advise FAO, WHO, and their Member States on the safety of food additives and contaminants and residues of veterinary drugs and pesticides in food. In addition, these committees serve as scientific advisory bodies to the Codex Alimentarius Commission, which is a subsidiary body of FAO and WHO. The primary objective of the Codex is to promote harmonization in the international trade of food commodities; it performs this task by establishing standards by consensus view that are based upon safety evaluations performed by JECFA and JMPR.

Most activities of the Codex Alimentarius Commission are carried out through commodity committees, general subject committees, and regional co-ordinating committees. JECFA and JMPR advise three general subject committees regard-

[1]International Programme on Chemical Safety, World Health Organization, 1211 Geneva 27, Switzerland.

ing the safety of food chemicals. These are the Codex Committee on Food Additives and Contaminants, or CCFAC, which is hosted by the government of The Netherlands, the Codex Committee on Pesticide Residues, or CCPR, also hosted by The Netherlands, and a new general subject committee, the Codex Committee on Residues of Veterinary Drugs in Foods, or CC/RVDF, which is hosted by the government of the United States of America. Special meetings of JECFA have been convened to evaluate veterinary drugs to advise CC/RVDF regarding the safety of their residues in food-producing animals.

This chapter will individually discuss the various types of food chemicals that are evaluated within the context of these scientific committees and the Codex, because intake data are used in different ways for each individual class of chemicals that is evaluated.

Food Additives

The primary endpoint of assessment of food additives by JECFA is the acceptable daily intake, or ADI. Usually it is expressed in numerical terms, but sometimes an "ADI not specified" is allocated. Such terminology is used for a food additive of very low toxicity which, on the basis of the available toxicological data and the total dietary intake of the substance arising from its use at the levels necessary to achieve the desired effect and from its acceptable background in food, does not, in the opinion of JECFA, represent a hazard to health [3].

Intake is not normally explicitly considered when establishing the ADI, as this endpoint is based on toxicological and biochemical data. However, when a substance is used as a food additive that is also naturally present in the diet, such as ascorbic acid, glutamic acid or nitrate, it is important to have some idea about its intake from natural sources [4]. Thus, under these conditions, JECFA requests intake information. The ADI that is established includes the total amount of the substance in food from all sources, unless the substance occurs in food in a chemical form different from that employed as a food additive. Intake information is also essential when considering whether an "ADI not specified" should be established. Before establishing such an endpoint, JECFA must be assured that the potential food additive uses of the substance will not lead to intake that will approach any numerical ADI that might be established based upon the toxicological data. Information that the Committee relies upon for making this determination includes the technological function of the additive, the types of foods in which it is likely to be used, and the maximum potential intake of such foods. Possible intake from other sources must also be kept in mind.

After JECFA has established an ADI for a food additive, Codex commodity committees may establish maximum levels for food additives in specific food items [5]. In most cases levels are set on the final product that is covered by the Codex Standard.

Proposed Codex Standards are referred back to CCFAC for acceptance of the food additive provisions that they contain. Thus, CCFAC serves as the clearinghouse for food additives in all Codex Standards. If there is cause for concern, potential intake is often considered when determining the suitability of a food additive provision. Thus, a survey of member governments has recently been performed on national regulations and results of intake studies on intense sweeteners in those countries [6]. Another recent example is a survey of the intake of several antioxidants by member governments, which was undertaken by CCFAC in 1987 [7] because JECFA had significantly changed the ADI values for some antioxidants at its thirtieth meeting in 1986. [8].

CCFAC is dependent upon survey data from member governments. This is indicative of the fact that Codex Standards do not include all the food additive uses approved in various countries and that food additives often are not used at the maximum levels permitted in the Codex Standards. Different methodologies are used in making these surveys, so direct comparison of results from different countries is sometimes difficult to make. In response to requests by a number of countries that have experienced difficulties performing such studies, CCFAC has developed guidelines for the simple evaluation of food additive intake [6]. The guidelines describe a stepwise approach to determine whether food additive intake exceeds the ADI allocated to a food additive. The first step is relatively easy and inexpensive, because it is based on the maximum authorized use. However, it is likely to result in a vast overestimate of intake. If this estimate results in intake below the ADI, then there is no need to expend further resources in estimating exposure. For those additives on which more refined estimates are required, further data should be developed, such as actual levels of additives in foods, rather than the maximum authorized use.

Food Contaminants

JECFA has evaluated a large number of food contaminants, including metals such as arsenic, cadmium, copper, lead, and tin. In most cases the databases are not sufficient for making definitive conclusions about the safety of the consequences of exposure to these substances; therefore, so-called provisional endpoints are set, with the understanding that as new significant data become available, re-evaluations will be performed. "Provisional maximum weekly intakes" (PTWIs) have been established for the majority of these substances. A weekly designation is used because these contaminants may accumulate within the body over a period of time. On any particular day, consumption of food containing above-average levels of the contaminant may exceed the proportionate share of its weekly tolerable intake. The assessment takes into account such daily variations, the real concern being prolonged exposure to the contaminant, because of its ability to accumulate within the body over a period of time [3]. An extreme example of this is cadmium, which is known to accumulate over most of the lifetime of a human being [9].

The usual 10-fold and 100-fold safety factors often cannot be used with food contaminants, because the level of exposure of at least some population groups is often high relative to observed toxicity. It is unrealistic to set PTWIs at levels so low that they are unattainable by a large proportion of the population. Therefore, JECFA considers intake data very carefully when evaluating food contaminants. GEMS (Global Environment Monitoring System)/Food provides information useful for this purpose. GEMS/Food also provides data to CCFAC for use in establishing guideline levels for contaminants in food commodities.

At its thirty-third meeting in March 1988 [9], JECFA re-evaluated methylmercury, at which time the Committee confirmed the PTWI of 3.3 µg/kg body weight. When setting this value, the Committee was aware that some species of fish contain levels of methylmercury of up to several parts per million, so that this value could be exceeded quite easily. However, JECFA did not make strong recommendations to limit the consumption of fish because of the fact that fish is nutritious and efforts are underway in many countries to increase fish consumption as an integral part of a well-balanced diet. Thus, the toxicity of contaminants must be balanced against the health impact of severely restricting intake of the foods in which they are present. These health impacts may include undernutrition and the lowered intake of essential nutrients. The Committee did recommend that efforts should continue to minimize human exposure to methylmercury that results from industrial exposure.

The chemical form of the contaminant is an important determinant of its toxicity. Inorganic arsenic was evaluated at the thirty-third meeting [9], at which time a PTWI of 0.015 mg/kg body weight was established. The primary source of inorganic arsenic is drinking water, and it was recognized that there is a need to reduce the arsenic intake of populations exposed to naturally elevated levels of inorganic arsenic in drinking water. On the other hand, data were reviewed that indicated that no ill effects were observed in population groups consuming fish containing organoarsenic resulting in organoarsenical intakes of as high as 0.05 mg/kg body weight per day (which is more than 20 times the PTWI for inorganic arsenic). This example highlights the need for identifying chemical species when performing intake studies.

With most of the contaminants that have been evaluated by JECFA, the primary route of exposure is through the diet. However, there are exceptions, as with inorganic arsenic, where the primary route of exposure is drinking water [9], and lead, where significant sources of exposure are the air, domestic environment (especially for children who may consume chips of lead-containing paint) and water [8]. The provisional tolerable intakes that are established by JECFA include exposure from all sources, so the significance of dietary intake must be considered in light of potential exposure from other sources.

As with food additives, Codex commodity committees recommend maximum levels of contaminants in those foods for which Codex Standards are being or have been established. These maximum levels are then ratified by CCFAC, taking into account intake levels derived from information gathered by GEMS/Food. CCFAC is also in the process of developing guideline levels for contaminants in food commodities other than standardized foods. These include aflatoxins, for which guideline levels in commodities such as cereals, milk and milk products, and animal feeds are being established, and certain food packaging materials [10]. The guideline levels take into account national regulations of member governments, the feasibility of the proposed limits, and dietary intake.

Pesticide Residues

JMPR consists of a FAO Panel of Experts on Pesticide Residues in Food and the Environment ("FAO Panel of Experts") and a WHO Expert Group on Pesticide Residues ("WHO Expert Group"). During the meetings the FAO Panel of Experts is responsible for reviewing pesticide use patterns, data on the chemistry and composition of pesticides and methods of analysis of pesticide residues, and for estimating the maximum residue levels (MRLs) that might occur as a result of the use of the pesticide according to good agricultural practices. The WHO Expert Group is responsible for reviewing toxicological and related data and for estimating, where possible, ADIs for the pesticides on the agenda.

The intake of pesticides is not usually explicitly considered by either group. Thus, the impact of the establishment of an MRL on intake of the pesticide is not considered. To make accurate estimates requires knowledge of (a) intake of the commodities on which MRLs are set and (b) actual residue levels of the pesticide on the commodity. The MRL represents the maximum level that should be present based on field trials that represent good agricultural practice; the actual level of residue normally present will almost always be less than the MRL.

CCPR uses the MRLs established by JMPR as the basis for "Codex MRLs." Sometimes questions are raised at CCPR as to whether the acceptance of Codex MRLs could result in a situation in which the ADI would be exceeded. Ordinarily this question can be answered with confidence only at the national or local level, because (a) diets vary widely from region-to-region and country-to-country, so dietary patterns within a country must be considered; (b) actual residue levels may be different in one country compared to another due, for example, to differing climatic conditions; and (c) Codex MRLs do not always represent all the commodities on which residues are permitted in a country.

GEMS/Food has prepared *Guidelines for Predicting Dietary Intake of Pesticide Residues* [11]. These Guidelines have been developed to describe procedures for predicting the dietary intake of pesticide residues, thereby assisting national authorities in their considerations regarding the acceptability of Codex MRLs.

The procedures used in these Guidelines start with the most exaggerated intake predictions and proceed toward more-and-more realistic ones. By starting with the most exaggerated intake predictions, it is possible to eliminate at an early stage those pesticides, of which the intakes are unlikely to exceed the ADI. This is the same approach used in the guidelines for the simple evaluation of food additive intake mentioned earlier.

Despite the fact that accurate determinations of intake cannot be made at the international level, it is the intention of the FAO and WHO Secretariats of JMPR to use the Guidelines to remove from further consideration those pesticides the intakes of which are not likely to exceed the ADI under exaggerated conditions. Participants in CCPR have also strongly encouraged this approach [12]. To this end, hypothetical global diets and information on correction factors that can be used for the edible portion of commodities and losses of residue on storage, processing, and cooking are being developed. This information will be used for making very crude estimates of intake at JMPR. More realistic estimates can only be made at the national level.

Veterinary Drug Residues

Two meetings of JECFA have been devoted exclusively to the evaluation of residues of veterinary drugs in food [13,14]. ADIs and Maximum Residue Levels in meat products have been established for some substances at these meetings.

At its third session, CC/RVDF [15] accepted the following draft definition of Maximum Residue Level:

Maximum Residue Level (MRL) is the maximum concentration of residue resulting from the use of a veterinary drug (expressed in mg/kg or µg/kg on a fresh weight basis) that is recommended by the Codex Alimentarius Commission to be legally permitted or recognized as acceptable in or on a food.

It is based on the type and amount of residue considered to be without any toxicological hazard for human health as expressed by the Acceptable Daily Intake (ADI), or on the basis of a temporary ADI that utilizes an additional safety factor. It also takes into account other relevant public health risks as well as food technological aspects.

When establishing an MRL, consideration is also given to residues that occur in food of plant origin and/or the environment. Furthermore, the MRL may be reduced to be consistent with good practices in the use of veterinary drugs and to the extent that practical analytical methods are available.

At its thirty-fourth meeting [14], JECFA agreed that this definition is essentially equivalent to the definition for Acceptable Residue Level that it had developed at its thirty-second meeting [13]. Henceforth, JECFA will use the term "recommended MRL" to differentiate its recommendations from those of the Codex.

The above definition makes clear that intake is an important consideration in establishing MRLs. For the purpose of calculating MRLs, the following daily intake values, which are considered to be upper-range values, are used: 300 g meat (muscle tissue), 100 g liver, 50 g kidney, 50 g tissue fat, 100 g egg, and 1.5 liters milk [14].

Operationally, JECFA proceeds as follows:

1. The substance is evaluated toxicologically and, if appropriate, an ADI is established.

2. The amount of residue expressed as parent drug equivalents is determined in various tissues sampled at selected withdrawal times.

3. The daily intake of residues, expressed as parent drug equivalents, is calculated based on the above intake figures. Corrections are made for the toxicological potency of the residues relative to the parent drug and the bioavailability of bound residues, if known.

4. The maximum daily intake of residues calculated in 3. is compared with the ADI (assuming an average adult body weight of 60 kg) to make sure that the intake does not exceed the ADI. If intake is below the ADI, then the residues determined in 2. go forward as "recommended MRLs." If intake exceeds the ADI, the residue levels must be reduced by, for example, increasing withdrawal times.

5. A prime requirement for a recommended MRL is that practical analytical procedures are available for measuring the residue at that level.

CC/RVDF is surveying governments regarding the intake of meat products [15]. The results of this survey may be useful for the purpose of establishing MRLs. However, in most cases it will probably not be necessary to use refined estimates of intake, because, even using the upper range intake figures cited above, calculated daily intakes will probably rarely exceed the ADI. The advantage of using a high intake estimate is that one does not have to be particularly concerned about which animal species contain residues of the drug. Thus, when one assumes that 300 g of muscle tissue is consumed per day, it does not matter whether it is beef or pork, because it is extremely unlikely that a person will consume 300 g of beef muscle tissue plus 300 g of pork muscle tissue in one day. When establishing recommended MRLs it is sufficient to base it simply on the meat product and not be concerned about the proportion that is beef and the proportion that is pork.

Summary

JECFA and JMPR have evaluated a large number of food additives, food contaminants, pesticide residues, and veterinary drug residues. These evaluations are used by the Codex Alimentarius Commission when establishing food standards for commodities moving in international trade. Evaluations performed by JECFA and JMPR are also used by FAO and WHO Member States for establishing national regulations.

Intake data are used in different ways for the different classes of substances evaluated by JECFA and JMPR, so they are considered separately. When evaluating the safety of food additives, intake data are explicitly considered only when establishing ADIs "not specified" and when evaluating food additives that are also naturally present in the diet. CCFAC performs surveys on food additives when there is concern that intake may exceed the ADI. To help governments estimate intake, CCFAC has developed guidelines for the simple evaluation of food intake.

Intake data are carefully considered by JECFA when evaluating food contaminants, because the level of exposure of at least some population groups is often high relative to observed toxicity. In some cases, the health benefit of limiting exposure to the contaminant must be balanced against the adverse impact of limiting the intake of a nutritious food.

The intakes of pesticides are not usually explicitly considered when JMPR establishes ADIs and MRLs. CCPR uses the MRLs established by JMPR as the basis for "Codex MRLs." Accurate estimates of intake cannot be made at the international level. However, to assist national authorities in their considerations regarding the acceptability of Codex MRLs, *Guidelines for Predicting Dietary Intake of Pesticide Residues* have been developed. These Guidelines are designed for use at the national level, but they will also be used to remove from consideration those pesticides the intakes of which are not likely to exceed the ADI under exaggerated conditions.

The estimation of intake is an integral component of recommended MRLs for veterinary drugs in meat products established by JECFA. The estimates of intake are exaggerated, which provides an extra margin of safety.

References

1. WHO (1957) General principles governing the use of food additives. First report of the Joint FAO/WHO Expert Committee on Food Additives. FAO Nutrition Meetings Report Series, no. 15, 1957; WHO Technical Report Series, no. 129, Rome and Geneva (out of print).
2. WHO (1962) Principles governing consumer safety in relation to pesticide residues. Report of a meeting of a WHO Expert Committee on Pesticide Residues held jointly with the FAO Panel of Experts on the Use of Pesticides in Agriculture. FAO Plant Production and Protection Division Report, no. PL/1961/11; WHO Technical Report Series, no. 240, Rome and Geneva.
3. WHO (1987) Principles for the safety assessment of food additives and contaminants in food. Environmental Health Criteria no. 70. WHO, Geneva.
4. WHO (1974) Evaluation of certain food additives. Eighteenth report of the Joint FAO/WHO Expert Committee on Food Additives. FAO Nutrition Meetings Report Series, no. 54, WHO Technical Report Series, no. 557, and corrigendum, Rome and Geneva.
5. FAO and WHO (1983) Food additives. Codex Alimentarius, Volume XIV. Rome and Geneva
6. Codex Alimentarius Commission (1989) Report of the twenty-first session of the Codex Committee on Food Additives and Contaminants. FAO, ALINORM 89/12A, Rome
7. Codex Alimentarius Commission (1987) Report of the nineteenth session of the Codex Committee on Food Additives. FAO, ALINORM 87/12A, Rome
8. WHO (1987) Evaluation of certain food additives and contaminants. Thirtieth report of the Joint FAO/WHO Expert Committee on Food Additives. WHO Technical Report Series, no. 751, Geneva
9. WHO (1989) Evaluation of certain food additives and contaminants. Thirty-third report of the Joint FAO/WHO Expert Committee on Food Additives. WHO Technical Report Series, no. 776, Geneva

10. Codex Alimentarius Commission (1988) Report of the Twentieth Session of the Codex Committee on Food Additives and Contaminants. FAO, ALINORM 89/12, Rome

11. WHO (1989) Guidelines for predicting dietary intake of pesticide residues. Prepared by the Joint UNEP/FAO/WHO Food Contamination Monitoring Programme in collaboration with the Codex Committee on Pesticide Residues. World Health Organization, Geneva

12. Codex Alimentarius Commission (1988) Report of the twentieth session of the Codex Committee on Pesticide Residues. FAO, ALINORM 89/24, Rome

13. WHO (1988) Evaluation of certain veterinary drug residues in food. Thirty-second report of the Joint FAO/WHO Expert Committee on Food Additives. WHO Technical Report Series, no. 763, Geneva

14. WHO (1989) Evaluation of certain veterinary drug residues in food. Thirty-fourth report of the Joint FAO/WHO Expert Committee on Food Additives. WHO Technical Report Series, No. 788, Geneva

15. Codex Alimentarius Commission (1988) Report of the third session of the Codex Committee on Residues of Veterinary Drugs in Foods. FAO, ALINORM 89/31A, Rome

CHAPTER 9

The Importance of Within-Person Variability in Estimating Prevalence

C.T. Sempos,[1] A.C. Looker,[1] C.L. Johnson,[1] and C.E. Woteki[1]

Introduction

There are four major uses of national nutrition data [1–3]:

1. Assessment and monitoring
2. Regulation
3. Evaluation of the impact of diet on the risk of disease or death
4. Commercial uses

All four require precise and accurate estimates of prevalence.

It is important for national health planning to know the percentage or prevalence with intakes above or below set criteria at any one point in time, as well as to have the ability to monitor trends over time. Furthermore, prevalence estimates are important to identify groups at greatest risk of nutritional deficiency, to develop and evaluate the effectiveness of government health policy which may include regulatory action, to estimate attributable risk and to aid in the development of foods and food products to meet consumer needs.

Since the first National Health and Nutrition Examination Survey (NHANES I) the National Center for Health Statistics has been conducting periodic national nutrition surveys in the United States (Table 9.1). A cornerstone of those surveys has always been the production of national estimates of the intake of individual foods, nutrient intake from those foods and the total nutrient intake by Americans. In October 1988, the latest survey, NHANES III went into the field. The primary dietary survey instrument in NHANES III, as in past NHANES, is the 24-hour recall [2].

Leaving aside the discussion of the accuracy of the various dietary survey methodologies and the nutrient estimation procedures associated with them [4–7], the single most important aspect affecting our ability to use NHANES data

[1]National Center for Health Statistics, 6525 Belcrest Road, Room 900, Hyattsville, MD 20782, USA.

Table 9.1. The National Health and Nutrition Examination Surveys (NHANES)

Surveys	Dates	Ages	Sample size
NHANES I	1971–74	1–74 years	28 043
NHANES II	1976–80	6 months–74 years	27 801
Hispanic HANES	1982–84	6 months–74 years	15 924
NHANES I Follow-up	1982–84	25–75 years	14 407
NHANES III	1988–94	2 months +	40 000

Source: NCHS, Division of Health Examination Statistics.

to make accurate national prevalence estimates is the within-person or intraindividual variation associated with dietary patterns. No matter how the dietary data are used the underlying assumption is, nearly always, that the intake estimates reflect the "usual" consumption patterns of individuals. A one-day record or a 24-hour recall, however, is not sufficient to describe an individual's "usual" intake of food and nutrients [8–10]. A great deal has been written about the effects of within-person variation on correlation coefficients and other measures of association [8–13], but very little of its effects on prevalence estimates [14–17].

This chapter discusses the following topics related to the estimation of prevalence in national nutrition surveys:

1. Ratios of within-person to between-person variation
2. Effects of within-person variation on the distribution of values in a population
3. Effects of within-person variation on prevalence estimates
4. How many replicate diet records are needed from each individual to obtain a reasonably accurate estimate of an individual's "usual" intake
5. The impact of within-person variability on the design of national nutrition surveys

Ratios of Within-Person to Between-Person Variation

There are two general ways to evaluate the impact of within-person variability. The first is merely to examine that variance estimate or its standard deviation. Such a value is useful for making clinical decisions about the number of repeated measurements of, say, serum total cholesterol that are necessary before reaching a treatment decision. The second is to evaluate the ratio of within-person to between-person variation (s^2_w/s^2_b). That ratio or its derivatives is used to evaluate the effect of within-person variation on correlation and regression coefficients [11–13] and on prevalence estimates [15,16].

A within-person to between-person ratio above one indicates that there is more variability within individuals than there is between them. A ratio of less than one indicates that there is more variability between individuals than within them.

Table 9.2. Variance components for women from Beaton et al. and from NHANES II (1976–80)

Variable	Beaton et al[a]			NHANES II[b]
	s^2_{w}[c]	s^2_{b}[c]	$s^2_{\mathrm{w}}/s^2_{\mathrm{b}}$	s^2_{obs}[c]
Cholesterol (mg)	47 002	10 858	4.3	58 537
Saturated fatty acids (% energy)	15.21	7.84	2.0	19.73
Calcium (mg)	85 849	94 249	0.9	262 754

[a]Adapted from Table 3 [12] and Table 4 [18].
[b]Women 45–54 years of age.
[c]s^2_{w} = within-person variance, s^2_{b} = between-person variance and s^2_{obs} = the total variance for the observed distribution.

Any ratio which is greater than zero will potentially result in biased prevalence estimates.

In general, the values of $s^2_{\mathrm{w}}/s^2_{\mathrm{b}}$ for nutrients are greater than one [8–12,15,16,18,19]. Values of $s^2_{\mathrm{w}}/s^2_{\mathrm{b}}$ for dietary cholesterol, saturated fatty acids as a percentage of total calories and dietary calcium are shown in Table 9.2; the values were calculated from data reported by Beaton et al. [12]. The values of the ratios shown for women in Table 9.2 are typical of the range of values for most nutrients. Ratios for vitamins A and B12 and fruits and vegetables high in vitamins A and C are generally much greater than four [8,9,15], although they are the exceptions. When nutrient intakes from vitamin-mineral supplements are included, ratio values for highly supplemented nutrients will decrease [8]. In contrast to ratio values for nutrients, ratios for serum analytes tend to be less than one with some exceptions [20–23]. But they are not zero. Although serum analytes and biochemical data are not discussed here such data are often collected as part of nutritional surveys. As a result, the implications for the design and analysis of national nutrition surveys, as will be discussed below, apply as well to the collection of serum data and to any physical measurement for which there is within-person variability.

Effects of Within-Person Variation on the Distribution of Values in the Population

As previously stated, the occurrence of significant "within-person," or intraindividual, variation in dietary nutrient intake of individuals is now well recognized, as is the need for several daily dietary records to estimate "usual" dietary intake of an individual [8–17]. Within-person variance has also been noted in biochemical measures of nutritional status, so that a measurement based on a single blood or urine sample may not be appropriate for estimating the "usual" circulating level of a nutrient for an individual [20–23]. Less well recognized,

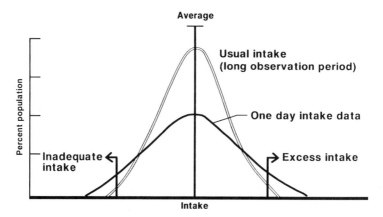

Figure 9.1. Effect of within-person variation on the distribution of observed nutrient intake values. (From Beaton [14].)

however, is the effect of within-person variance on the distributions of dietary intakes or biochemical measures from groups or populations when based on a single measurement. Although means or medians for groups may be adequately estimated from single measurement, within-person variance can distort estimates of the centiles above or below the mean by increasing the total variance of the distribution, which makes the distribution flatter and wider [14–16]. Thus, prevalence estimates based on a single day's intake from a 24-hour recall or diet record along with estimates based on single blood draw will be overestimates of both the "prevalence of 'inadequate' or 'excess' intakes in the population" [14]. Fig. 9.1 clearly illustrates the problem.

A frequent response to Fig. 9.1 after shock and dismay is disbelief. The argument goes something like this: "Common sense says that even if there is within-person variation all that should happen is that some individuals will have relatively high values others will be relatively low which should all balance out and as a result there should be no effect on the distribution of values." Statistical theory often agrees with common sense, but in this instance this does not, unfortunately, appear to be the situation.

The total variance (s^2_{obs}) of the observed distribution is the sum of the between-person (s^2_b) and within-person (s^2_w) variances [24] as described in Equation 1

$$s^2_{obs} = s^2_b + s^2_w/k \qquad (1)$$

where k is the number of replicate measures obtained from each individual. As shown in the equation, the only way to diminish the impact of s^2_w on s^2_{obs} is by increasing the number of replicate measures (k). The effect cannot be diminished by increasing the sample size.

Rearranging Equation 1 shows the relationship between the ratio of the standard deviation in the total population to the standard deviation for the between-person variation (s_{obs}/s_b) and s_w/s_b [16].

$$s^2_{obs}/s^2_b = (s^2_b + (s^2_w/k))/s^2_b = (1 + s^2_w/s^2_b(k))$$

$$s_{obs}/s_b = (1 + s^2_w/k(s^2_b))^{1/2} \tag{2}$$

Equation 2, again, points out that if s^2_w is greater than zero the value under the radical will be greater than one as will be the ratio of s_{obs}/s_b. Ideally the standard deviation of the observed distribution will be equal to the interindividual standard deviation $(s_{obs} = s_b)$. For dietary variables, though, this is rarely the case.

Effects of Within-Person Variation on Prevalence Estimates

The effect of within-person variation on dietary cholesterol, saturated fatty acid and dietary calcium distributions of 45–54-year-old women from NHANES II $(n = 763)$ was examined by comparing the shape of the distribution curves before and after the distributions were "adjusted" to remove the within-person variation. NHANES II was chosen because it is the source of the most recent NHANES dietary data.* Those three nutrients were chosen because they are good examples of nutrients which are important risk factors for the development of coronary heart disease in the case of cholesterol and saturated fatty acids, and, of (possibly) osteoporosis in the case of calcium.

It was also decided to use the data for women because the range of values for s^2_w/s^2_b is typical of dietary data (Table 9.2) [16]. They go from a relatively high value of 4.3 for cholesterol to a relatively common value of 2.0 for saturated fatty acids and a relatively low value of 0.9 for calcium.

An approach developed by the US National Academy of Sciences Subcommittee on Criteria for Dietary Evaluation [15] was used to adjust the distributions of the three nutrients to remove the within-person variation. Each individual's value for the nutrients was adjusted using the following formula:

$$\text{Adjusted value} = \bar{x} + (x_i - \bar{x})(s_b/s_{obs}) \tag{3}$$

where $\bar{x}$ is the average or group mean, and where x_i is the value for the ith participant. The ratio s_b/s_{obs} can either be obtained by taking the inverse of the result from Equation 2 or by dividing s_b from Beaton's data by the observed standard deviation for the sample distribution of, say, women aged 45–54 years

---

*Parenthetically, it should be noted that all the estimates in this paper are unweighted estimates. That is, they were not weighted to produce national estimates and the prevalence estimates given here should not be construed as national estimates. Because the variance components produced, so far, are based on very small sample sizes it is not felt that they can be used to produce national estimates. Accordingly, the results given herein are only examples of how variance components could be used to adjust for within-person variability.

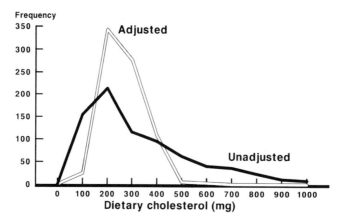

Figure 9.2. Dietary cholesterol intake for women 45–54 years of age from NHANES II (1976–80).

($n = 763$). In the latter case, the adjusted distribution would be standardized to the s_{obs} of the sample distribution from, for instance, NHANES II. For this chapter the calculation was performed using the former method.

The observed and adjusted distributions for the three nutrients are shown in Figs. 9.2–9.4. As in Fig. 9.1, the unadjusted distributions are flatter and wider than the adjusted ones. Notice that on moving from cholesterol with a high value for s^2_w/s^2_b to calcium with a relatively low value for s^2_w/s^2_b the effect within-person variability on the distributions is diminished. But even for calcium, there is still considerable flattening and widening of the distribution.

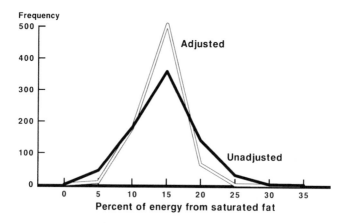

Figure 9.3. Saturated fatty acid intake for women 45–54 years of age from NHANES II (1976–80).

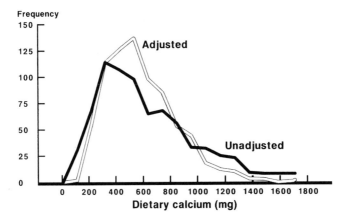

Figure 9.4. Dietary calcium intake for women 45–54 years of age from NHANES II (1976–80).

Equation 3 does not affect the mean of the distribution; only the shape of the distribution. It forces $s_{obs} = s_b$. An example of the calculation of s_b/s_{obs} from Equation 2 for cholesterol (Table 9.2) is:

$$s_{obs}/s_b = (1 + 4.3/1)^{1/2} = (5.3)^{1/2} = 2.30$$

$$s_b/s_{obs} = 1/2.30 = 0.435$$

In these calculations $k = 1$; that is, the ratio s_b/s_{obs} for the situation in which only a one-day dietary record or 24-hour recall was collected.

To demonstrate the bias associated with prevalence estimates attributable to within-person variability and to demonstrate the importance of an appreciation of that bias to survey planning, the "true" prevalences and the observed and predicted prevalences for the raw or unadjusted data were calculated. The prevalence value from the adjusted distribution was taken as the "true" prevalence. The observed prevalences were taken from the raw unadjusted data for the same cut points. The cut off values used to define the prevalence of abnormal values in the adjusted and unadjusted distributions were: > 300 mg for cholesterol; <10% of energy intake (kcal) from saturated fatty acids; and >800 mg for calcium.*

---

*When using tables of areas under a standard normal distribution it is usually easier to compute the z-value or percentage for the smallest portion of the curve. That percentage, or in this case prevalence, for the smallest portion may not, however, represent the group at risk. This is the situation for saturated fatty acids and it may also be for calcium [25,26]. For saturated fatty acids estimates are determined of the prevalence with intakes < 10% and for calcium the prevalence > 800 mg. Subtract from one the value from the table or areas to obtain the at risk population in such circumstances.

Table 9.3. "True," predicted and observed prevalence estimates together with the number of repeated measurements needed to reduce the observed prevalence to within 5% of the "true" prevalence. Data for women 45–54 years of age from NHANES II (1976–80)

Variable	Prevalence (%) "True"	Predicted	Observed	Number of repeated measurements[a]
Cholesterol				
> 300 mg	15	33	37	39
Saturated fatty acids				
< 10%	15	27	22	18
Calcium > 800 mg	12	20	21	9

[a]Values calculated from the formula $(1 + s^2_w/s^2_b(k))^{1/2}$ where s^2_w = within-person variation, and s^2_b = between-person variation [16].
Sources: Ratios of s^2_w/s^2_b, Beaton et al. [12,18]; Intake data, NCHS, NHANES II (1976–80).

To calculate the predicted prevalences for the unadjusted distribution or raw data, the "true" prevalence values are converted into a z-value for the predicted prevalence by dividing the z-value for the "true" prevalence by s_{obs}/s_b

$$z\text{-value (predicted prevalence)} = \frac{z\text{-value ("true" prevalence)}}{s_{obs}/s_b} \qquad (4)$$

As stated above, s_{obs}/s_b was calculated from Equation 2 using Beaton's [12,18] variance ratios. Finally, the z-value for the predicted prevalence is converted into the predicted prevalence using the table of areas under the normal curve.

Dietary cholesterol is a nutrient with a relatively large variance ratio. If it is assumed that the "true" prevalence of cholesterol intakes > 300 mg percent is 15% the predicted prevalence would then be 33%. In the original raw data an observed prevalence of 37% was found which is very similar to the predicted value (Table 9.3). Turned around, if the within-person variation is removed from the raw distribution, the prevalence would drop from 33% to 15%. Note the large differences between the observed or predicted prevalences and the "true" values. These differences represent the effect of removing the within-person variation.

For both saturated fatty acids and dietary calcium the "true" value is approximately half the observed and predicted values (Table 9.3). Again, in both cases the predicted prevalence is reasonably close to the observed one. In a recent study using iron status indicators, close agreement was also found between the observed and predicted prevalence [23]. The results from that study and those reported here suggest the importance of using estimates of s^2_w/s^2_b to "remove" the effects of within-person variation from distributions of both dietary and biochemical variables.

How Many Replicate Measures are Needed?

It is possible to estimate the number of replicate records necessary to remove the effect of within-person variation from a distribution using Equation 2. To obtain

Table 9.4. Ratios of observed standard deviation to between-person standard deviation[a]

s^2_w/s^2_b	Number of replicate measurements				
	1	2	3	5	10
1.0	1.41	1.22	1.15	1.10	1.05
2.0	1.73	1.41	1.29	1.18	1.10
4.0	2.24	1.73	1.53	1.34	1.18

[a]Values calculated from the formula $(1 + s^2_w/k(s^2_b))^{1/2}$ where s^2_w = within-person variation and s^2_b = between-person variation (reference [16], Table 5, p 45).

prevalence estimates for cholesterol that are within 5% of the "true" value approximately 39 one-day food records or 24-hour recalls would have to be collected (Table 9.3). For calcium, even though the variance ratio is relatively low, nine one-day food records or 24-hour recalls would be required!

The Impact of Within-Person Variability on the Design of National Nutrition Surveys

Obviously very few studies will have the time and the resources to collect more than a few replicate records. But even two dietary records or 24-hour recalls can significantly reduce the bias in the prevalence estimates due to within-person variability (Table 9.4).

Another option would be to collect at least two dietary records or recalls from a random sample of participants. Their replicate data could then be used to estimate both s^2_w and s^2_b. With those values and s^2_{obs} from the total sample it would be possible to use Equation 3 to produce prevalence estimates which were adjusted to remove the within-person variance [16].

The variance ratios for food and nutrients, as stated above, are generally greater than one. The variance ratios for serum analytes, although they are usually less than one, are not zero. Accordingly, when planning a study, investigators should take into account the amount of within-person variability present in the nutrient or blood analyte of interest and, at a minimum, should consider obtaining replicate samples from a random sample of the study population in order to adjust the distribution of the entire group.

Postscript

In NHANES III, two replicate 24-hour recalls will be collected at 4 and 8 months after the first one for all participants aged 50 years and older at baseline. Funding sources do not allow the collection of multiple records for all participants. A 5% sample, over the entire age range, will, however, have a second examination which will include both a 24-hour recall and a blood draw. From this replicate data it is hoped to get representative values of s^2_w/s^2_b which will allow production of prevalence estimates that are much closer to the "true" prevalences.

References

1. Murphy RS, Michael GA (1982) Methodologic considerations of the National Health and Nutrition Examination Survey. Am J Clin Nutr 35:1255–1258
2. Woteki CE, Briefel RR, Kuczmarski R (1988) Contributions of the National Center for Health Statistics. Am J Clin Nutr 47:320–328
3. Yetley EA, Hanson EA (1983–4) Data sources and methods for estimating consumption of food components. J Toxicol Clin Toxicol 21:181–200
4. Burk MC, Pao EM (1976) Methodology for large-scale surveys of household and individual diets. Home Economics Research Report No. 40. Agricultural Research Service. United States Department of Agriculture. Washington, DC
5. Becker BG, Indik BP, Beeuwkes AM (1960) Dietary intake methodologies – a review. University of Michigan Research Institute, Ann Arbor
6. van Staveren WA, Burema J (1985) Food consumption surveys: frustrations and expectations. Naringsforskning 29:43–52
7. Sampson L (1985) Food frequency questionnaires as a research instrument. Clin Nutr 4:171–178
8. Sempos CT, Johnson NE, Smith EL et al. (1985) Effects of intraindividual and interindividual variation in repeated dietary records. Am J Epidemiol 121:120–130
9. Sempos CT, Johnson NE, Smith EL et al. (1986) Estimated ratios of within-person to between-person variation in selected food groups. Nutr Rep Int 34:1121–1127
10. Basiotis PP, Welsh SO, Cronin FJ et al. (1987) Number of days of food intake records required to estimate individual and group nutrient intakes with defined confidence. J Nutr 117:1638–1641
11. Liu K, Stamler J, Dyer A et al. (1978) Statistical methods to assess and minimize the role of intraindividual variability in obscuring the relationship between dietary lipids and serum cholesterol. J Chron Dis 31:399–418
12. Beaton GH, Milner J, Corey P et al. (1979) Sources of variance in 24-hour dietary recall data: implications for nutrition study design and interpretation. Am J Clin Nutr 32:2546–2559
13. Jacobs DR Jr, Anderson JT, Blackburn H (1979) Diet and serum cholesterol. Do zero correlations negate the relationshipo: Am J Epidemiol 110:77–87
14. Beaton GH (1982) What do we think we are estimating. In: Beal VA, Laus MJ (eds) Proceedings of the symposium on dietary data collection, analysis and significance. Research Bulletin No. 675, pp 36–48. Massachusetts Agricultural Research Station, University of Massachusetts, Amherst, MA
15. National Research Council, Subcommittee on Criteria for Dietary Evaluation (1986) Nutrient adequacy: assessment using food consumption surveys. National Academy Press, Washington, DC, 146 pp
16. Anderson SA (ed) (1986) Guidelines for use of dietary intake data. Life Sciences Research Office. Federation of American Societies for Experimental Biology. Bethesda, MD, 90 pp
17. Anderson SA (1988) Guidelines for use of dietary intake data. J Am Dietet Assoc 88:1258–1260

18. Beaton GH, Milner J, McGuire V et al. (1983) Sources of variance in 24-hour dietary recall data: implications for nutrition study design and interpretation. Carbohydrate sources, vitamins and minerals. Am J Clin Nutr 37:986–995

19. McGee D, Rhoads G, Hankin J et al. (1982) Within-person variability of nutrient intake in a group of Hawaiian men of Japanese ancestry. Am J Clin Nutr 36:657–663

20. Harris EK, Kanofsky P, Shakarji G et al. (1970) Biological and analytical components of variation in long-term studies of serum constituents in normal subjects. Clin Chem 16:1022–1027

21. Tangney CC, Shekelle RB, Raynor W et al. (1987) Intra- and interindividual variation in measurements of β-carotene, retinol and tocopherols in diet and plasma. Am J Clin Nutr 45:764–769

22. Looker A, Woteki C, Sempos C et al. (1989) Limitations in existing nutrition survey methods. In: Livingston G (ed) Nutritional status assessment of the individual. Food and Nutrition Press, Trumbull CT, pp 57–67

23. Looker AC, Sempos CT, Liu K et al. (1990) Within-person variance in biochemical indicators of iron status: effects on prevalence estimates. Am J Clin Nutr (in press) 52:541–547

24. Neter J, Wasserman W (1974) Applied linear statistical models. Richard D. Irwin, Homewood, IL, p 53

25. Expert Panel (1988) Report of the National Cholesterol Education Program Expert Panel on detection, evaluation and treatment of high blood cholesterol in adults. Arch Intern Med 148:36–69

26. National Institutes of Health Consensus Conference (1984) Osteoporosis. JAMA 252:799–802

CHAPTER 10

Use of Food Composition Data Banks in Nutrient Intake Studies

M. Ahola[1]

Introduction

The compatibility and limitations of food composition data and nutrient data banks have been addressed and discussed at international level on several occasions [1–4]. Several loose organizations such as EUROFOODS in Europe [2], NORFOODS in the Nordic countries [5] and the global organization INFOODS [1] have been established to promote national and international participation and co-operation in this area. Their main goal has been to link together the compilers, and users, as well as the analysts of food composition data in order to facilitate communication. The aim has also been to be concerned with the quality of food composition data and to create general guidelines for the production, management and use of food composition data [6].

The approach of this chapter is mainly that of a nutritionist carrying out dietary surveys although several other professional groups also need food composition data. Nutrition research strategies/study design for dietary surveys have become more and more complex. This has led to a demand for more items to be included in the nutrient data banks. Interest is focused not only on new nutrients but also on non-nutrient substances. Therefore, it is desirable to hold data on additives, contaminants, allergens etc. and even radionuclides, in addition to data on bioavailability of some nutrients mainly those foods of greater importance in human nutrition.

The quantitative assessment of the nutritional value of the diet depends on information on the composition of foods combined with food consumption. The methodology of dietary assessment suffers from a low scientific status and a variable level of subjectivity [7]. Therefore, a lot of effort has been put in to study the validity and representativeness of dietary assessment methods. However, an equally important aspect in carrying out a dietary survey is the quality of the food composition data which are needed in order to calculate the dietary intake. The validity of results obtained in dietary surveys is greatly dependent on the reliabil-

[1]The Finnish Foreign Trade Association, P.O. Box 908 SF-00101 Helsinki, Finland

ity of data on the nutritional composition of the foods consumed. Biases in food composition data and their effects on nutrient intake have rarely been discussed by nutritionists.

Uses of Food Composition Data

Food consumption can be measured at different levels of the food supply chain, creating a need for including compositional data at the corresponding level in the database. Measurements at the wholesale commodity level of the foods form the basis of "Food Balance Sheet" studies and require data at this level together with estimates of potential losses in the food chain. Measurements at the "Household Budget" level require retail, as purchased, data. The nutrient data bank for studies of individual food consumption should cover data for foods and mixed cooked dishes and have an extensive selection of nutrients and non-nutrients [8].

In any nutrient intake study, in addition to the study population (individual, group and national levels) the dietary intake method selected (24-hour recall, dietary history, weighing method, food recording techniques, the food frequency questionnaire) determines the level (aggregation level of food items) of the nutrient data bank. For those who are not familiar with dietary surveys the process of collection of food consumption data is briefly described here using the 24-hour method as an example. In this method, respondents are asked to report all foods and beverages consumed on the previous day. Each food item is coded and identified by name, including brand names if appropriate, whether it was raw, dry or frozen, how it was prepared, and for mixed dishes having no code, the major ingredients are asked. After this the food composition database is used to calculate the nutrient contents of the foods. When using for instance the 24-hour recall method or food recording techniques the aggregation level of foods is very low. People are able to remember or to make notes quite accurately even by a brand name, on what they have eaten. Therefore, the nutrient data bank has to be organized on a detailed level including exact data on a large selection of foods and dishes.

When using the dietary history method where a study period may be, for instance a year, many more rarely consumed dishes and foods have to be merged. A self-administered food frequency questionnaire is a simple and quick method which is sometimes used to measure the intake of a certain nutrient such as vitamin C. In this case the questionnaire is designed to contain a wide range of foods and dishes which are a good source of vitamin C in a study population. Only the vitamin C intake is calculated combining food frequency data with the data on vitamin C composition of consumed foods. For this, vitamin C values and vitamin C losses of the data bank have to be checked in particular.

In up-dating the data bank and planning new analysis projects it is preferable to concentrate on those foods that make the greatest contribution to total nutrient intake.

Demand for and Problems of Food Composition Data Available

Nutritionists are mostly interested in foods as consumed in a certain country or a region. They need food composition data on raw ingredients, processed foods, foods for special nutritional uses, baby foods etc. New foods are continually being developed and offered to the consumers. Many traditional foods can now be made using different and new ingredients, and so they may have significantly different nutritional composition. Composition data available on novel foods (snacks, sweets, health foods) is rather incomplete. Foods differ genetically and environmentally. Nutritional content of foods is also affected by the ways in which they are produced, handled, processed and prepared. No table or database is able to contain all this information but the user has to modify the database for his or her own purposes.

The number of food components suggested as being of interest grows rapidly. In total only a small amount of the foods usually consumed have been analyzed. Comprehensive analytical research projects on some nutrients such as The Mineral Element Study in Finland [9], are seldom conducted on a representative sample of the national foods. Frequently the food composition values inserted in a data bank are of variable quality because they have been collected from different sources: from laboratories of research, control and manufacture, other food composition tables etc. Very often there are no analysis data for a specific food or nutrient and the user has to fill in gaps with imputed (estimations based on similar foods or nutrients), calculated (values derived from recipes by calculation) or borrowed (values taken from other tables or databases without reference to the original source) values or if no data are available, mark the value absent [6,10].

Only some countries have so-called national nutrient data banks where the quality of the bank is carefully controlled and documented by experts. The most common practice is for institutes or single researchers to compile their own databases according to their needs. In these cases there exists a danger that the contents are incompatible even within a country. The main limitation of these databases has been the lack of resources for updating the food composition data, and for keeping up a continuous know-how concerning every aspect needed in the maintenance of a valid, high quality database.

Factors to be Taken into Account in Compilation of the Nutrient Database

Food composition tables and nutrient databases/banks vary in the manner the data have been collected. Some tables are based on direct collection of the foods consumed in the country; other tables are based on a compilation of published and unpublished sources from the international literature; some tables just copy values from other tables. Tables also differ in the way they convert nitrogen into protein, in the way they define carbohydrates and in the way they calculate the metabolizable energy provided by proteins, fats, carbohydrates and alcohol [7].

The purpose here is not to give comprehensive advice on how to compile a nutrient data bank. Southgate and Greenfield [6] give guidelines for the production and management of food composition data. However, some essential factors in using and compiling nutrient data bases are emphasized here.

Quality of Food Composition Data

When using food composition data the user has to be aware of the origin of the nutrient data. Major food tables routinely contain data on 50–100 food components. In addition, there are many nutrients which have biological activity but there are no acceptable analytical methods for determining their levels in a given food sample. Inconsistencies and incompatibilities between data sets arise because foods analysts often use different methods for analyzing the same food component. As a consequence there is great variation in single nutrient values [11]. Few analyses have been carried out for several rare components. Thus, the user is confronted by the fact that satisfactory analyses can never be available for each component of each food desired and the gaps have to be filled by using imputed, calculated and borrowed values instead of having no data at all.

The fixed nutrient value offered by most tables, and desired by most users, is most often misleading. The amount of a nutrient in a food has a statistical distribution and cannot be adequately represented by the result of a single analysis or by the average of analyses performed. A number of factors, both systematic and unsystematic, influence the levels of nutrients and other compounds in different products. The composition of milk, and thus also the composition of butter, varies regularly between winter and summer [12]. In some food composition tables the range (Danish tables) or standard error (US tables) is given. That is not, however, user-friendly for a nutritionist.

A nutritionist does not welcome missing values for any component of food, because this leads to underestimations of the "true" nutrient intake. But borrowing the value from tables of other countries can be dangerous. Rimestad et al. [13] gives examples of this by calculating the selenium and iron intakes of an average Norwegian household by using Norwegian and Finnish data on selenium and iron composition [9,14]. Selenium intake of the household was 18 µg/day using Finnish values and 86 µg/day using the Norwegian values. The iron intakes were 13.3 mg/day and 10.6 mg/day, respectively. In addition the situation in Finland has changed completely because all agricultural multinutrient fertilizers have been supplemented with selenium since 1983. The average Finnish selenium intake in 1984 was 39 µg and in 1986 92 µg/10 MJ (38.3 ng/kcal) [15].

When comparing Nordic food composition tables several dissimilarities in the food composition have been found due to different food standards, food fortification and supplementation, meat cutting practices, cattle breeding policy and soil composition.

Nomenclature and Food Grouping

An important problem in using nutrient databases is the identification of individual products (brand names, local synonyms, foods with same name but different content). Nutritionists should be able to obtain and code the nutrient values correctly and quickly. An unambiguous nomenclature, proper food grouping, and practical coding system would increase the utilization of food composition data. All these issues have been discussed internationally [16,17].

Recipe Calculation

Food composition data are not available for all the various preparation methods and all possible combinations of industrially and home-made foods that may be consumed because analyses of dishes are rather expensive. Therefore, calculation of recipes has been used. Recently, the problems in the recipe calculation (food yields, nutrient losses and gains) have been discussed extensively, for example by Bergström [18] and Powers and Hoover [19]. Although large amounts of data are currently available to support the calculation methods, more data are needed to supply information for the vast array of preparation and cooking procedures indicated on recipes. However, the amount of additional data needed could be minimized if a single general purpose method was designated as the preferred calculation method [19].

Documentation

Documentation of the nutrient figures in food composition tables and databases is considered necessary. In most modern food composition tables, a reference value is documented for each separate nutrient value. Missing values are also separated from real zero values [20,21].

Conclusion

The usefulness of the nutrient data used is considerably enhanced if the nutrient values obtained are representative for foods as consumed. Great attention has to be given to the evaluation of the food composition data. Guidelines for the quality of food composition data and data banks, nomenclature of food items, and food grouping which make the coding phase easier and comparisons possible are needed as well as the international guidelines for corrections or factors which are appropriate for different nutrients and food preparation techniques.

In order to avoid the pitfalls of food composition, the existing networks of compilers, analysts and users of food composition tables and nutrient databases, such as INFOODS, EUROFOODS and NORFOODS, are important. Also the compilation of national or regional data bank systems where the quality of the compositional data is evaluated, is recommended to save resources and to aim towards compatibility of data banks. However, the user has to remember that a nutrient data bank is never a ready-made entity but it has to be modified according to the study design.

References

1. Rand WM, Young VR (1984) Report of a planning conference concerning an international network of food data systems (INFOODS). Am J Clin Nutr 39:144–151
2. West CE (ed) (1985) EUROFOODS: towards compatibility of nutrient data banks in Europe. Ann Nutr Metab 29 (suppl 1):1–76
3. Rand WM, Windham CT, Wyse BW, Young VR (eds) (1985) Food composition data: a user's perspective. Report of a conference held in Logan, Utah, USA, 26–29 March 1985. The United Nations University, Tokyo
4. Fox K, Stockley L (eds) (1988) EUROFOODS. Proceedings of the second workshop. Food Sci Nutr 42F:1–82
5. Bergström L (1984) Översikt av NORFOODS' verksamhet 1982–1984. Vår Föda 36:325–329
6. Southgate DAT, Greenfield H (1988) Guidelines for the production, management and use of food composition data: an INFOODS project. Food Sci Nutr 42F:15–23
7. Hautvast JGAJ, Klaver, W (eds) (1982) The diet factor in epidemiological research. EURONUT report 1. Wageningen, 154 pp
8. Southgate DAT (1988) Database requirements for studies of food and nutrient consumption. Proposals of CEC support for database required for executing various types of study on food consumption. Towards improved data on food consumption in Europe. (Abstract). CEC-Agrofoods/Eurofoods Workshop, Brussels, 15–16 June
9. Koivistoinen P (ed) (1980) Mineral element composition of Finnish foods. Acta Agriculturae Scandinavica, Stockholm, (suppl 22), 171 pp
10. Meyer B, van Oosten-van der Goes HJC, van Staveren WA, West CE (1988) Missing values in European food composition tables and nutrient data bases: preliminary results of a survey. Food Sci Nutr 42F:29–34
11. Hollman PCH, Katan MB (1985) Report of the Eurofoods interlaboratory trial 1985 on laboratory procedures as a source of discrepancies between food tables. RIKILT Report 85.67, Wageningen, 85 pp
12. Bruce Å, Bergström L (1983) User requirements for data bases and applications in nutrition research. Food Nutr Bull 5:24–29
13. Rimestad AH, Ahola M, Bergström L, Möller A, Reykdal O (1988) Naeringsmiddeltabeller - bruk og utarbeidelse. Näringsforskning 32:26–32
14. Rimestad AH (1984) Innholdet av selen, kopper, sink og magnesium i en del matvarer. Matvett 4:1–4
15. Varo P, Alfthan G, Ekholm P, Aro A (1988) Selenium intake and serum selenium in Finland: effects of soil fertilization with selenium. Am J Clin Nutr 48:324–329
16. Arab L, Wittler M, Schettler G (1987) European food composition tables in translation. Springer, Heidelberg
17. Truswell AS (1988) INFOODS progress on nomenclature of foods. Food Sci Nutr 42F:24–28
18. Bergström L (1988) NLG project (nutrient losses and gains in the preparation of foods) report 1985. Food Sci Nutr 42F:8–12

19. Powers PM, Hoover LW (1989) Calculating the nutrient composition of recipes with computers. J Am Diet Assoc 89:224–232
20. Möller A (ed) (1989) Levnedsmiddeltabeller. Statens Levnedsmiddelinstitut. Storkökkencentret, levnedsmiddelstyrelsen, 864 pp
21. Rastas M, Seppänen R, Knuts L-R, Varo P (eds) (1989) Nutrient composition of foods. Publications of the Social Insurance Institution. Karisto, Hämeenlinna, 452 pp

CHAPTER 11

National Surveillance of Food and Contaminant Intake: The Danish Experience

J. Højmark Jensen[1,2] and A. Møller[1]

In 1983 The National Food Agency established a food monitoring system in order to follow the content of nutrients and contaminants in foods in a systematic manner. When the data from this system are combined with the results from the national food consumption survey from 1985 it is possible to calculate the intake by the participants of both nutrients and contaminants. Also, it is possible to make an estimate of the maximum intake of food additives. Calculations like these are used as a basis for regulating food fortification and the use of food additives as well as establishing safe levels for the content of contaminants in foods.

The National Food Consumption Survey

In 1985 the National Food Agency of Denmark carried out a nationwide food consumption survey [1,2]. The objectives of the survey were:

- To identify population groups which are at risk from a nutritional point of view
- To evaluate the significance of fortifying foods with nutrients
- To estimate the exposure of different population groups to contaminants and food additives
- To identify foods which contribute significantly to the nutrient intake in different population groups
- To contribute to studies of the relationship between diet and health/diseases

The survey included 2242 persons, 15–80 years of age. They constituted a representative sample of the adult Danish population. The participants in the survey were interviewed about their food consumption habits using a dietary history method, which was developed particularly for this survey.

[1]The National Food Agency of Denmark, Mørkhøj Bygade 19, DK-2860 Søborg, Denmark.
[2]Present address: Flæsketorvet 75, 1711 København V, Denmark.

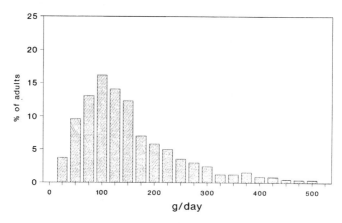

Figure 11.1. Potatoes: daily intake.

The dietary history method gives information about the usual diet of an individual during an extended period of time. There is no doubt, that the method tends to overestimate regularity in the eating pattern. The method itself encourages the participants in the survey to emphasize the usual food consumption, because it is easier to remember the usual meal pattern than all the unusual events that have interfered with the habitual food intake. The results of the survey are, however, in excellent agreement with the results from other similar data sources, such as food balance sheets, household budget surveys, and other food consumption surveys. The conclusion is that the average consumption found in the survey is very close to the real average intake except for a few foods and beverages, such as sugar and alcohol.

The dietary history method used in the present survey enables the ranking of individuals according to their intake of foods, nutrients, contaminants and other

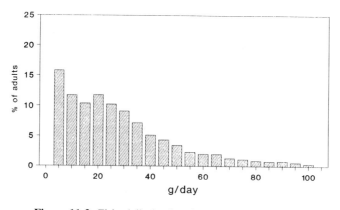

Figure 11.2. Fish: daily intake of cooked edible portion.

known constituents of food. The absolute level of intake has, however, to be used with caution. Moreover, we do not know the degree of uncertainty.

The Food Intake

The distribution in the intake of potatoes and fish within the adult population is shown in Figs. 11.1 and 11.2. The shape of the intake curve for potatoes is typical of foods that are consumed by practically everybody. These foods are cereals, white bread, rye bread, coarse vegetables, meat, poultry, separated fats and eggs. Figure 11.2 illustrates the shape of the intake curve for foods and beverages that are consumed by some people only, for instance cheese, soft drinks, beer and tea.

Table 11.1. The food monitoring system 1983–1987

Food category	Nutrients	Trace elements and nitrate	Pesticides and PCB
Fruit and vegetables	Fat, protein, ash, dry matter, fiber, vitamin C (tomatoes: glutamic acid)	As, Cd, Cr, Hg, Ni, Pb, Se In vegetables also nitrate	
Cereal products	Fat, protein, ash, dry matter, vitamins B1 and B6, fiber, Ca, Fe, K, Mg, Na, Zn	As, Cd, Cr, Hg, Ni, Pb, Se	
Dairy products and eggs	Fat, protein, ash, dry matter, fatty acids, vitamins A, B1 and B2, Ca, Fe, K, Mg, Na, Zn and J	As, Cd, Cr, Hg, Ni, Pb, Se Only in eggs	DDT, dieldrin, HCB, α-HCH, β-HCH, lindane (γ-HCH), heptachloroepoxide, PCB
Fish	Fat, protein, ash, dry matter, fatty acids, vitamin D	As, Cd, Cr, Hg, Ni, Pb, Se	DDT, dieldrin, HCB, α-HCH, β-HCH, lindane (γ-HCH), heptachloroepoxide, PCB
Meat	Fat, protein, ash, dry matter Beef, chicken, pork: Fe, Mg, Zn, vitamins B1, B2 and B6		
Offal	Fe, fat, protein, ash, dry matter	As, Cd, Cr, Hg, Ni, Pb, Se	
Animal fat			DDT, dieldrin, HCB, α-HCH, β-HCH, lindane (γ-HCH), heptachloroepoxide, PCB

The Food Monitoring System

The contents of both nutrients and contaminants in foods on the Danish market have been analyzed by the National Food Agency and associated laboratories for several decades.

In 1983 a food monitoring system was established. It is designed to supply data on the changes over time in the contents in foods of nutrients and contaminants. It is also designed to be linked with the data from the food consumption survey in order that the nutrient and contaminant intake of the population can be calculated.

The food monitoring system covers nutrients as well as heavy metals/other trace elements, nitrate, pesticides and PCB in selected foods. The compounds/ substances are selected on the basis of the existing knowledge about their nutritional importance or toxicity, their occurrence in foods, and the actual consumption of these foods. Table 11.1 shows the elements of the food monitoring system for 1983–1987. In the first 5-year period approximately 10000 samples were analyzed. The results are stored in the food composition data bank of the National Food Agency.

The Intake of Substances from Foods

The Agency has developed a computer program that allows the data from the food consumption survey to be combined with the data from the food composition data bank. Therefore computation of the intake levels of nutrients and contaminants of the individuals who participated in the food consumption survey gives an idea about the distribution of intakes within the adult population.

Nutrients

Figs. 11.3–11.5 are examples of the results of the calculations on the nutrient level.

Fig. 11.3 illustrates how the fat-energy-% of the diet of Danish women and men is distributed. The fat-energy-% seems to be very high when compared to the recommended level of 30% of the dietary energy from fat. In fact almost all Danish adults seem to eat a diet that is higher in fat than the recommendations.

Fig. 11.4 indicates that a very large percentage of Danish women and men get more vitamin A than the recommended level of 800 and 1000 µg/day respectively.

Fig. 11.5 shows that the same is not the case for iron. The iron intake of most women in Denmark seems to fall below the recommended level of 12–18 mg/day.

The results regarding nutrient intakes have for instance been used to evaluate the nutritional importance of the fortification of foods. As a result of this evaluation the obligatory fortification of flour and margarines with vitamins and

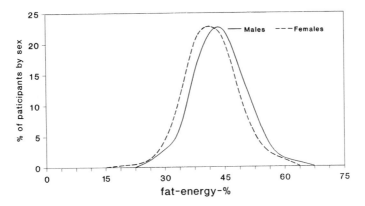

Figure 11.3. Percentage of dietary energy from fat.

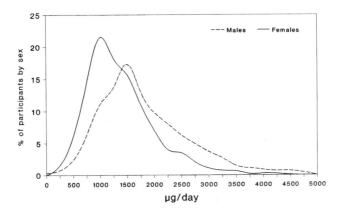

Figure 11.4. Daily intake of vitamin A.

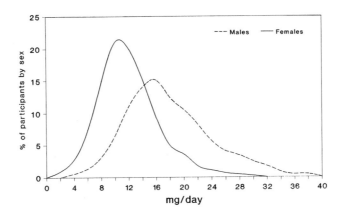

Figure 11.5. Daily intake of iron.

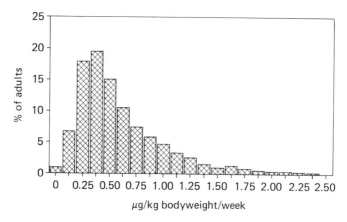

Figure 11.6. Weekly intake of mercury (PTWI: 3.3 μg/kg body weight per week).

minerals was abolished in 1987, because the contribution of the fortification to the total nutrient intake was either negligible or unnecessary.

Contaminants

Figs. 11.6–11.9 show the calculated intakes from foods of mercury, cadmium, lead and arsenic. For mercury, cadmium and lead it appears that the intakes from foods are well below the provisional tolerable weekly intake (PTWI) proposed by JECFA [3,4].

For arsenic the total intake of organic and inorganic arsenic is shown in Fig. 11.9. This cannot be compared to the PTWI value of 15 μg/kg body weight, since

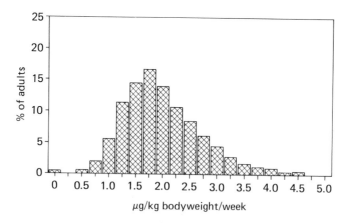

Figure 11.7. Weekly intake of cadmium (PTWI: 7 μg/kg body weight per week).

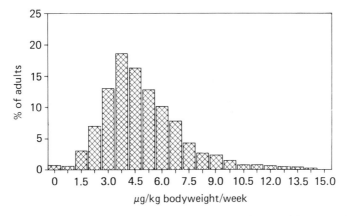

Figure 11.8. Weekly intake of lead (PTWI: 50 μg/kg body weight per week).

this value applies to inorganic arsenic only. Most of the arsenic in the Danish diet stems from fish. It is organic and probably less toxic than inorganic compounds. Arsenic is not considered to be a problem in Danish foods.

So far it has not been possible to calculate the exposure of the population to pesticides and organic pollutants from foods in the same manner as for heavy metals. The analyses of pesticide residues in foods have been concentrated on those foods where high contents are most likely. There are too many gaps in our knowledge about the content in other foods to allow us to make a calculation of the total exposure of the participants in the survey to pesticides from foods.

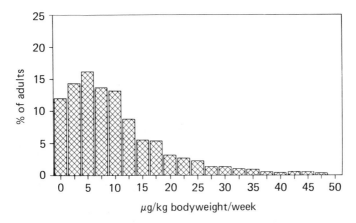

Figure 11.9. Weekly intake of total arsenic (PTWI (inorganic): 15 μg/kg body weight per week).

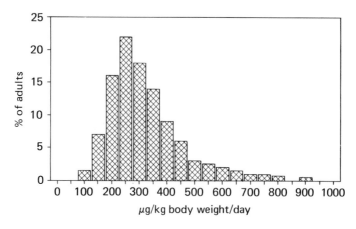

Figure 11.10. Maximum erythrosin intake (ADI: 50 µg/kg body weight per day).

Food Additives

The use of food additives in Denmark is regulated by the National Food Agency through the so-called positive-list [5]. The list specifies the maximum amount of a food additive that can legally be used in individual foods. Although the maximum amount of food additives that might be used is known, there is no complete picture of the actual use by the food industry. Therefore, no calculation can be made of the actual exposure of the population to food additives, but only an estimate of the maximum exposure, which would occur, if the food producers used all the permitted food additives in their maximum amounts. The calculated exposure will in all cases be higher than the actual, since most foods are manufactured without making full use of all permitted additives. The calculated maximum intake is, however, of considerable interest from a regulatory point of view. It allows a check to be made as to whether the limitations that have been introduced in the use of additives to individual foods are realistic in relation to the ADI-values.

Figs. 11.10 and 11.11 show, for instance, the intake distribution of the calculated maximum intakes of erythrosin and benzoic acid/benzoates. From the figures it appears that while the maximum intake of benzoic acid/benzoates permitted according to the positive-list is well below the ADI-value, the same is not the case for erythrosin. For erythrosin, however, the ADI-value has been reduced from 625 to 50 µg/kg body weight per day [4] very recently. The distribution curve in Fig. 11.10 has to be compared to the higher value of 625, since the lower ADI-value was not reflected in the positive-list at the time of the survey.

These calculations have proved that the method used to determine the amounts of food additives permitted in the "positive-list" is applicable. The method is the so-called budget-method [6]. It is not a scientific method, but a practical administrative tool to predict the maximum intake of a food additive. The main assump-

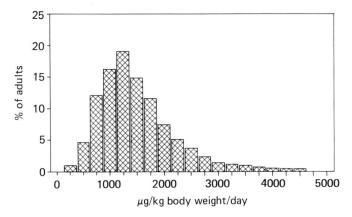

Figure 11.11. Maximum benzoic acid/benzoates intake (ADI: 5000 µg/kg body weight per day).

tion in the budget-method is that the maximum daily consumption for an adult is 1.5 kg of foods and 6 liters of beverages and water. It is also assumed that only half the foods are industrially processed and thus contain food additives. As far as the liquid intake is concerned the assumption is made that only 25% are beverages containing food additives. The ADI can be divided between solid and liquid foods according to technological needs. If the required level is too high compared to the ADI available the additive may be limited to either solid or liquid foods or to certain groups of foods.

The calculations show that each of these assumptions is reasonable for 90% of the adult population. The type of calculations illustrated in Figs. 11.10 and 11.11 confirm that the budget-method is a reliable tool in the administration of food additives.

References

1. Haraldsdottir J, Holm L, Jensen JH, Møller A (1986) Danskernes kostvaner 1985, 1. Hovedresultater, Levnedsmiddelstyrelsen, Søborg, Denmark, publication no. 136
2. Haraldsdottir J, Holm L, Jensen JH, Møller A (1987) Danskernes kostvaner 1985, 2. Hvem spiser hvad? Levnedsmiddelstyrelsen, Søborg, Denmark, publication no. 154
3. FAO/WHO (1972) Sixteenth report of the Joint FAO/WHO Expert Committee on Food Additives. WHO Technical Report Series no. 505, Geneva
4. FAO/WHO (1989) Thirty-third report of the Joint FAO/WHO Expert Committee on Food Additives. WHO Technical Report Series no. 776, Geneva
5. National Food Agency (1988) Fortegnelse over godkente tilsaetningsstoffer til levnedsmidler. Levnedsmiddelstyrelsen, Søborg, Denmark, publication no. 171
6. Hansen SC (1979) J Food Protect 42:429–434

CHAPTER 12

Experience of GEMS/Food in Coordinating Dietary Intake Studies

H. Galal-Gorchev[1]

The Joint UNEP/FAO/WHO Food Contamination Monitoring Programme, or GEMS/Food, forms part of the Global Environment Monitoring System established by the United Nations Environment Programme. GEMS is a collective effort to monitor the world environment in order to protect human health and preserve essential natural resources.

One of the objectives of GEMS/Food is to compile and analyze food contamination data on a global basis; the others are to improve and harmonize measurement methodologies among countries, increase the validity and accuracy of measurements, and support countries in their efforts to strengthen national food contamination monitoring programs. At present 37 countries participate in GEMS/Food. Each participating country submits data on the concentrations of agreed contaminants in individual foods and in total diets.

Nineteen contaminants are covered by GEMS/Food, including selected organochlorine pesticides such as DDT, aldrin, dieldrin, organophosphorus pesticides, such as malathion and parathion, PCBs, lead, cadmium, mercury and aflatoxins [1,2].

Measurements of contaminants in total diet provide the best estimates of human exposure and of the potential risks to health, if any. The risks to consumers are evaluated by comparison with toxicologically acceptable intake levels–ADIs or PTWIs (Acceptable Daily Intake and Provisional Tolerable Weekly Intake).

Information on contaminants in total diets has been collected by GEMS/Food since 1980. Information recorded includes the mean, median and 90th percentile values. In 1988 a total of 22 countries (mostly developed countries) were providing total dietary intake data to GEMS/Food. The composition of the diet, preparation for analysis, total weight of the diet and study approach vary widely from country to country. For instance, the amount of food consumed may be purposely exaggerated (3.3 kg/day) in order to protect extreme consumers; drinking water

[1]International Programme on Chemical Safety, Division of Environmental Health, World Health Organization, 1211 Geneva, Switzerland.

and alcoholic beverages may or may not be included in the diet; foods may not be cooked prior to analysis; the number of foods analyzed can vary from 10 to over 100; and finally, the type of study can be a market basket, a duplicate portion or a study of individual staple foods. Because of such differences, while trends within a country may at times be established, comparisons between countries should be done with caution.

In addition to actual dietary intake studies, estimates of intake of contaminants by the breast-fed infant may be obtained from the concentration of contaminants found in human milk. For the first three months of life, an infant consumes on average 120 g/day of human milk/kg of body weight. By multiplying the µg/kg concentration of a contaminant in human milk by 0.12, the approximate intake of the contaminant in µg/day/kg of body weight may be estimated and this in turn may be compared to the toxicologically acceptable intake level. Alternatively, an "acceptable level" of a contaminant in human milk may be computed by dividing the toxicologically acceptable intake by 0.12. Exceeding such intakes may not necessarily mean a health concern since toxicologically acceptable intakes are usually developed on the basis of lifetime exposure, whereas intake of contaminants from human milk is limited to a few months in a lifetime [3].

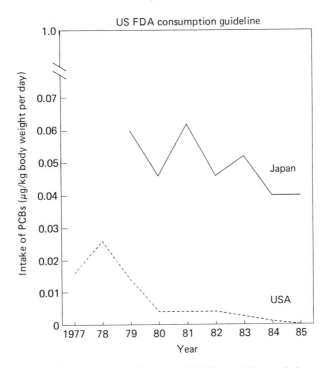

Figure 12.1. Average daily intake of PCBs – adult population.

Polychlorinated biphenyls (PCBs)

No tolerable intake level for man has been established by the Joint FAO/WHO Expert Committee on Food Additives (JECFA). The United States Food and Drug Administration has suggested a consumption maximum of 1 µg/kg body weight per day for adults.

Relatively few countries report dietary intake of PCBs. The consumption of fish and dairy products are the major contributing factors to the intake of PCBs. This is illustrated in Fig. 12.1 where intake of PCBs in Japan (with fish consumption averaging 90 g/capita/day) is appreciably higher than in the USA where fish consumption is about 20 g/capita/day. A decreasing trend in PCB intake is noted in the data from Japan.

Substantially higher daily intakes reported by New Zealand are due primarily to the high PCB intake from dairy products. In this case, the mean daily intake of 0.9 µg/kg body weight for the adult female approaches the FDA-suggested consumption maximum of 1 µg/kg body weight/day.

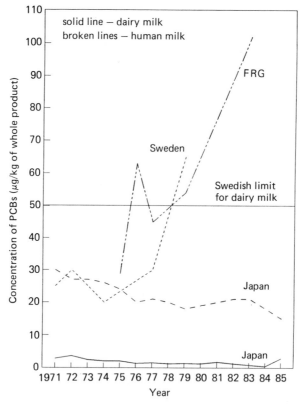

Figure 12.2. Median levels of PCBs in dairy milk (continuous line) and human milk (broken lines).

Estimates of intake of PCBs by the breast-fed infant may be obtained from human milk data. With a concentration of PCBs in human milk above 8 μg/kg, the intake of the breast-fed infant may exceed the advice given by FDA. As shown in Fig. 12.2, many of the concentrations reported are substantially above 8 μg/kg.

Lead

In 1972, JECFA established a PTWI for lead of 50 μg/kg of body weight, applicable to adults only. Because of the special concern for infants and children, in 1986 JECFA evaluated the health risks of lead in this population group and established a PTWI of 25 μg/kg of body weight.

Information on the dietary intake of lead is available from 19, mostly developed countries. Trends in intakes are shown for some of the countries in Fig. 12.3. It appears that a downward trend in lead intake has taken place in several countries. In some countries, this downward trend coincides with the period of conversion from lead soldered to non-lead soldered cans and during the phasing out of lead in petrol. With few exceptions, median and/or mean weekly intakes for average adults in several countries are less than 50% of the PTWI (Fig. 12.4).

Based on data from several countries, higher adult dietary lead intake occurs in

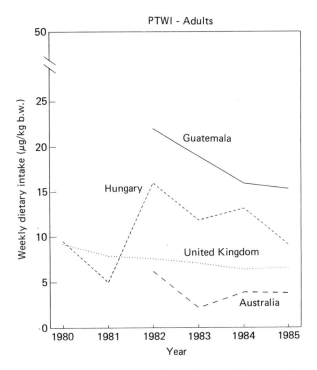

Figure 12.3. Median weekly dietary intake of lead – adults.

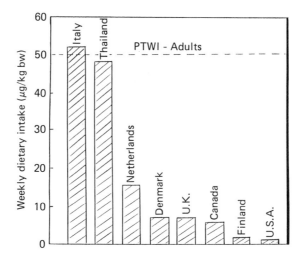

Figure 12.4. Mean intake of lead – adults.

industrial areas, in areas of high traffic density, in areas with high lead concentration in tap water, with higher consumption of wine or canned food, and can then approach or exceed the PTWI.

Relatively few countries report dietary intake of lead by infants and children. Selected data for infants and children up to four years of age are presented in

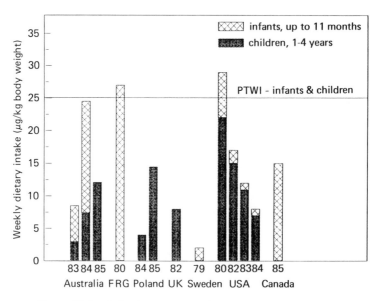

Figure 12.5. Median/mean intake of lead – infants and children.

Fig. 12.5. Since the PTWI of lead for infants and young children refers to the maximum intake from all sources of ingestion, the median/mean intakes should be well below 25 µg/kg body weight, because they may ingest lead from dust or soil. A reduction in lead intake by infants and children apparently occurred in the USA. There is possibly an increasing trend in lead intake for the 2-year old in Australia from 1983 to 1985. The lowest intake is reported in the 1979 study in Sweden for infants who are breast-fed.

Mean levels far in excess of the PTWI (in the 100 µg/kg body weight/week range) were obtained in studies carried out in the Federal Republic of Germany and the United Kingdom in areas with high lead content in tap water. This increase in dietary lead results from the water added to dehydrated infant formulas and infant cereals as well as the water which is consumed directly.

Cadmium

In 1988, JECFA established a PTWI of cadmium of 7 µg/kg body weight, applicable to adults as well as infants and children. The PTWI was derived from estimated accumulation over a period of 50 years at an exposure rate equivalent to 1 µg/kg body weight/day for adults; excursions above this figure may therefore be tolerated provided that they are not sustained for long periods of time.

No particular time trend was noticeable for countries submitting information over several years (Fig. 12.6). Average adult intake in different countries over the period 1980–85 are given in Fig. 12.7. Recent data submitted by Finland indicate that in this country the weekly intake of cadmium is approximately 1 µg/kg body weight.

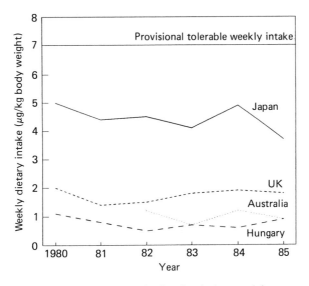

Figure 12.6. Dietary intake of cadmium – adults.

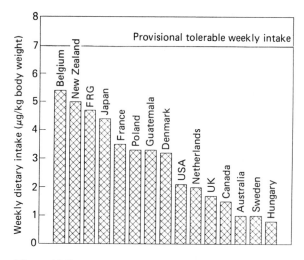

Figure 12.7. Average cadmium intake, adults, 1980–1985.

In many of the reporting countries, the median or mean cadmium intakes of adults constitute an appreciable percentage of the PTWI. Where the 90th percentile levels are reported, they approach or exceed the PTWI in some cases. Populations living in industrial areas have higher cadmium intake than those in non-industrial areas. High cadmium levels are found in animal kidney and molluscs. In Belgium it was noted that once-a-week consumption of mussels or kidney would result in a mean intake that would approximate the PTWI. Similarly, in Denmark, above average consumption of ox kidney, mussels from contaminated water or wild mushrooms would yield intakes that exceed the PTWI.

Cadmium intakes by infants increase appreciably with increasing concentration of cadmium in drinking water and may exceed the PTWI. However, such high intakes do not necessarily represent a health risk, provided that they are not sustained for long periods. Intake of cadmium by the breast-fed infant is low, indicating the lack of accumulation of cadmium in human milk.

Exposure to cadmium in the diet is of public health concern. It should continue to be monitored and appropriate measures taken to decrease it. Caution should be observed in consuming animal organs and shellfish from areas of known cadmium contamination.

Mercury

JECFA established a PTWI for the general population of 5 µg/kg body weight for total mercury, of which no more than 3.3 µg/kg body weight should be in the form of methylmercury. The Committee further noted that pregnant women and nursing mothers are likely to be at greater risk from the adverse effects of methylmercury.

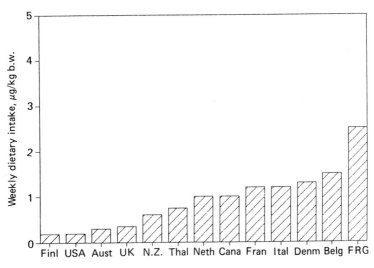

Figure 12.8. Mean intake of mercury – adults.

Mean weekly intake of total mercury for average adults are presented in Fig. 12.8; all intakes are below the PTWI.

The contribution of fish to the total dietary intake of mercury varies in different countries from 20% to 80%. The general assumption that fish is the main contributor to the intake of mercury may therefore at times not be justified.

The contribution of various foods to the total intake of a contaminant depends, of course, on the quantity consumed, and the contaminant concentration in that food. For instance, in the Netherlands a higher concentration of mercury is found in fish than in other foods. However, because of the relatively high consumption of grain and meat, the contribution of each of these two food groups to the total intake are about the same as that from fish, approximately 20% each. Similarly, in the Federal Republic of Germany, intake was approximately the same on days with and without fish consumption, indicating that fish was not the main source of mercury intake. As demonstrated in a UK study, the most highly exposed population groups are those living in coastal areas receiving discharges high in mercury (high fish consumption and high level of contamination).

Ensuring that the PTWI established by JECFA is not exceeded may be achieved through various options: advice on fish consumption, including choice of fish species and/or size; frequency of fish meals; establishment of standards which limit the mercury concentration in all seafood or in selected species; the banning or limitation of fishing in certain areas; limitation of anthropogenic sources of pollution that lead to higher methylmercury levels in fish. "Member States have to choose from these or any other possibilities, evaluating the efficacy, costs and benefits of alternative actions for each of the specific situations" [4,5].

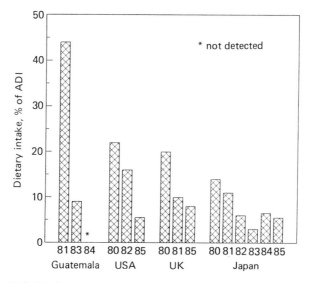

Figure 12.9. Median or mean dietary intake of aldrin plus dieldrin by adults.

Organochlorine Pesticides

As shown in Fig. 12.9, average daily intake of aldrin plus dieldrin by adults has declined in countries reporting to GEMS/Food. For the remainder of the organochlorine pesticides studied (DDT, heptachlor, lindane, endrin and endosulfan), intakes seldom exceed 1% of the respective ADI. The restrictions or bans imposed on use in some if not most of the reporting countries account for these low intakes.

Organophosphorus Pesticides

Reported intake of diazinon, fenitrothion, parathion and parathion-methyl are less than 1% of the respective ADIs, and in the majority of cases these compounds are not detected in total diet studies.

References

1. WHO/UNEP (1987) GEMS. Global pollution and health–results of health-related environmental monitoring. WHO/UNEP, Geneva
2. UNEP/FAO/WHO (1988) GEMS. Assessment of chemical contaminants in food. UNEP/FAO/WHO, Geneva
3. WHO (1985) The quantity and quality of breast milk. WHO, Geneva

4. UNEP/FAO/WHO (1980) Draft report of meeting of experts on environmental quality criteria for mercury in Mediterranean seafood (UNEP/MED - HG/14). UNEP/FAO/WHO, Geneva
5. UNEP/FAO/WHO (1983) Assessment of the present state of pollution by mercury in the Mediterranean sea, and proposed control measures (UNEP/WG. 91/5). UNEP/FAO/WHO, Athens

Part III
Actual Intake Versus Potential Intake in Relation to Nutritional and Safety Standards

CHAPTER 13

Macronutrient Intake in Relation to Nutritional Standards

J.A.T. Pennington[1]

Since there appears to be no precise definition for the term "macronutrient," a somewhat liberal interpretation has been made in this chapter to include discussion of protein, fat, digestible carbohydrate, dietary fiber and alcohol (Table 13.1). The macronutrients are distinguished from the micronutrients (vitamins and minerals) by their greater abundance in the food supply and by the fact that, except for dietary fiber, they provide energy. Macronutrients are also used for the growth, maintenance, or regulation of body tissue.

Dietary intakes of some or most of the macronutrients are traditionally assessed from national food consumption surveys. As a reference point, Table 13.2 presents data on the intake of macronutrients from the United States Department of Agriculture (USDA) 1985 Continuing Survey of the Food Intake of Individuals (CSFII) [1]. These data represent 24-hour recalls from 658 men and 1459 women 19–50 years of age.

The standards against which macronutrient intakes may be compared include recommended intakes and dietary guidelines. Most countries have developed recommended daily nutrient intake standards for specified age-sex groups. These recommended intakes are sufficient to maintain health and protect against the consequences of nutrient deficiency. For example, in the US there are recommended allowances for energy and protein [2]. Some countries also have dietary guidelines which suggest dietary practices to encourage adequate nutrient intake and decrease the risk of diet-related diseases. The Dietary Guidelines for Americans [3] provide non-quantitative suggestions with regard to intake of energy and most of the macronutrients including fat, saturated fat, cholesterol, starch, dietary fiber, sugar and alcohol (Table 13.3). The Surgeon General's Report on Nutrition and Health [4] supports and exemplifies these guidelines by providing a detailed summary of the scientific literature concerning the relationship of diet to various diseases. A recent, comprehensive report from the Committee on Diet and Health of the Food and Nutrition Board, National Academy of Sciences [5]

[1]Associate Director for Dietary Surveillance, Center for Food Safety and Applied Nutrition, US Food and Drug Administration, Washington, DC 20204, USA.

Table 13.1. The macronutrients

Proteins (including polypeptides and amino acids)
Fats (lipids)
Glycerides (mono-, di-, and tri-)
Saturated fatty acids
Monounsaturated fatty acids
Polyunsaturated fatty acids
Cholesterol
Digestible carbohydrates
Starches
Sugars (mono- and disaccharides)
Dietary fiber
Alcohol (ethanol)

provides suggested levels of intakes for most of the macronutrients. These suggested levels are shown in Table 13.2 together with the average intakes of adults in the US.

Protein

Functions and Effects of Deficiency

The consequences of protein deficiency are well known and, in the extreme, are manifested as protein-calorie malnutrition (PMC), especially in children and

Table 13.2. Average and suggested intakes of macronutrients for adults in the US

	(Females/males)			
	Average intakes[a]		Suggested intakes[b]	
Energy	82/94	% REI	2000/2700	kcal/day
Protein	144/175	% RDA	44/56	g/day
Total fat	37/36	% of kcal	≤ 30	% of kcal
Saturated fat	13/13	% of kcal	< 10	% of kcal
Polyunsaturated fat	7/7	% of kcal	< 10	% of kcal
Cholesterol	304/435	mg/day	< 300	mg/day
Digestible carbohydrate	46/45	% of kcal	≥ 55	% of kcal
Dietary fiber	12/18	g/day	20–30, but < 35	g/day
Alcohol			< 1	oz/day

[a]Average intakes are from Human Nutrition Information Service [1].

[b]Suggested intakes for energy and protein are the Recommended Energy Intakes (REI) and Recommended Dietary Allowances (RDA) [1], respectively, for a 55-kg woman and a 70-kg man. Suggested intakes for total fat, saturated fat, polyunsaturated fat, cholesterol, digestible carbohydrate, and alcohol are based on recommendations of the National Academy of Sciences [5]. Suggested intakes for dietary fiber are based upon recommendations of the National Cancer Institute [68].

Table 13.3. Dietary guidelines for Americans [3]

Eat a variety of foods
Maintain desirable weight
Avoid too much fat, saturated fat, and cholesterol
Eat foods with adequate starch and fiber
Avoid too much sugar
Avoid too much sodium
If you drink alcoholic beverages, do so in moderation

other vulnerable groups in poor countries or pockets of poverty within wealthier countries. Protein is required for the growth and maintenance of body tissues. Many body tissues and substances (e.g., skin, hair, nails, muscle, bone, hemoglobin, certain hormones, enzymes, antibodies, connective tissue) are adversely affected when protein intake is inadequate. Symptoms of protein deficiency include poor growth, anemia, fatigue, muscle wasting, multiple nutrient deficiencies (from decreased absorptive capacity of gastrointestinal cells), changes of skin, hair, and nails, failure of wounds to heal, delayed and impaired tooth development, osteoporosis, and decreased immune function.

Effects of Excess

Protein intake has traditionally been low in poor countries and more than adequate in wealthier countries. Recommended intakes for protein in the US are 44 g/day for women and 56 g/day for men [2], and average intakes are 63 and 98 g/day [1] (144% and 175% of the recommended allowance) for women and men, respectively. On a body weight basis, the recommended allowance for protein is 0.8 g/kg [2] and the National Academy of Sciences [5] suggests that intakes should not exceed 1.6 g/kg. Average protein intakes in the US are 1.1 g/kg for women and 1.4 g/kg for men.

Amino acids consumed in excess of body need are deaminated and either burned for fuel or converted into body fat. There are, however, some concerns about the health effects of excess protein in the diet.

1. There is some evidence that blood cholesterol may be affected by the amount and type of protein in the diet [6]. The substitution of vegetable protein for animal protein in the diets of hyperlipidemic patients resulted in decreased serum cholesterol [7,8]; however, the relationship of dietary protein to serum cholesterol is confounded by the level and type of fats in the diet [4,5].

2. Associations between the consumption of animal protein and the incidence of certain cancers has been observed in several epidemiologic studies [9–13]. Several studies show associations between meat consumption and cancer [14,15]. However, the association between cancer and protein intake is also confounded by high correlations between protein and fat intakes [4,5].

3. High protein intakes may cause bone loss by increasing calcium excretion in the urine [16,17].

4. High protein diets may contribute to the decline in renal function which occurs after the fourth decade of life. Increased glomerular capillary blood flow and pressure associated with high protein diets may contribute to progressive renal injury in certain individuals [18,19].

5. Synthesis of brain neurotransmitters serotonin, dopamine and norepinephrine depends on the levels of tryptophan (precursor for serotonin) and tyrosine (precursor for dopamine and norepinephrine) in the blood and hence in the diet. Pharmacologic amounts of tryptophan have been given to induce sleep [20,21], to relieve anxiety and suppress food consumption [22], and to relieve pain [23,24]. Tyrosine has been used in the treatment of Parkinson's disease [25,26] and endogenous depression [27]. These uses of tryptophan and tyrosine require further confirmation.

Protein and Amino Acids: Special Problems

1. Products of amino acid and protein metabolism, some of which are toxic, accumulate during kidney failure. Dietary protein restriction minimizes toxicity and retards renal failure in a variety of renal diseases. Unfortunately, no dietary therapy prevents protein wasting in severely ill patients with acute renal failure [28–30]. Giving large amounts of amino acids to such patients increases formation of urea and may lead to uremic poisoning or a more frequent need for dialysis treatments.

2. Food allergies result from absorption of intact (undigested) proteins from offending food(s). The body reacts to the protein allergen with antigen–antibody reactions. The allergic symptoms may include malaise, fever, diarrhea, headache, fatigue, and rashes. Common allergy-producing foods include milk, eggs, wheat, oranges, fish, shellfish, chocolate, tomatoes, strawberries, corn, and peanuts. Treatment requires identification and avoidance of the offending food(s).

3. Celiac disease (also known as non-tropical sprue or gluten-induced enteropathy) is a genetic, immunologic reaction to the gluten fraction of proteins from wheat, rye and oats. For patients with this disorder, gluten causes atrophy of cells that line the small intestine. This results in malnutrition, stunting of growth, and anemia. Strict removal of gluten from the diet alleviates the symptoms and restores the integrity of the intestinal mucosa.

4. Phenylketonuria (PKU), an inborn error of metabolism, results from lack of the hepatic enzyme phenylalanine hydroxylase, which converts the amino acid phenylalanine into tryptophan. High levels of phenylalanine and its metabolites increase in the blood and urine. This disease results in damage to the neurological system and leads to hyperactivity, convulsive seizures, and mental retardation. PKU can be detected at birth by a simple blood test. It requires a phenylalanine-restricted diet throughout infancy, childhood, and adolescence. Foods sweetened

with aspartame should not be consumed by persons with PKU, and women who have this disease should not breastfeed their babies.

5. Other less-common inborn errors of metabolism involving amino acids include maple syrup urine disease, homocystinuria, leucine-sensitive hypoglycemia, and histidinemia.

Fats

Functions and Effects of Deficiency

The principal function of dietary fat is to contribute to body energy needs. A small quantity of linoleic acid, an essential fatty acid, is required for maintaining the exterior surface membrane of body cells and for initiating primary and secondary antibody response [31]. Deficiencies of essential fatty acids are rarely seen, but have resulted in poor growth, liver abnormalities, and eczematous skin lesions in infants.

Effects of Excess

The recommendations of the National Academy of Sciences [5] suggest that total fat not exceed 30% of energy intake, that saturated fatty acids be less than 10% and polyunsaturated fatty acids be less than 10% of energy intake, and that cholesterol not exceed 300 mg/day. The US diet contains about 36%–37% of energy from fat, 13% of energy from saturated fat, 7% of energy from polyunsaturated fat, and 300 (women) and 435 (men) mg of cholesterol/day [1]. Problems associated with excessive fat intake include obesity, coronary heart disease (CHD) and some cancers. Other more questionable associations with high fat intake include hypertension, formation of cholesterol gallstones, impaired immune function, and multiple sclerosis.

1. The formation of *atherosclerotic lesions* in coronary arteries is increased in proportion to levels of total and low density lipoprotein (LDL) cholesterol in blood, which in turn are increased by diets high in total and saturated fat, but decreased by diets containing polyunsaturated and/or monounsaturated fat [4]. There are strong associations between intake of fat, especially saturated fat, and elevated blood cholesterol levels, atherosclerosis, and CHD [4]. Intervention to lower elevated blood cholesterol levels has been shown to reduce CHD risk and to slow lesion progression [4]. The effect of dietary cholesterol on blood cholesterol is somewhat weaker and more variable than that for dietary saturated fatty acids [4].

Arterial thrombosis is induced by vascular injury and the response of blood platelets, and platelet reactivity is associated with the fatty acid composition of the diet [4]. Replacement of dietary saturated fat with polyunsaturated vegetable oils is associated with decreased platelet aggregation and clotting activity

[32,33]. Increased dietary intake of linoleic acid (the precursor of prostaglandins that regulate platelet aggregation and thrombogenesis) has been associated with significant reductions in platelet aggregability [34,35].

The fatty acids in fish and other marine animals are rich in long-chain polyunsaturated fatty acids of the omega-3 series and may assist in reducing CHD mortality [36–38] by reducing triglyceride and very low density lipoprotein (VLDL) levels [39–42].

2. Death rates for *cancers* of the breast, colon, and prostate are directly proportional to estimated dietary fat intakes [43,44]. Other cancers that have been related to fat intake are those of the rectum [9], ovaries [45] and endometrium [46]. A worldwide correlation between breast and colon cancer mortality and total fat consumption has been demonstrated [47].

3. An increased intake of polyunsaturated fatty acids may be associated with *lower blood pressure* [48–51]. Blood pressure change might be mediated through changes in prostaglandin metabolism caused by increased intake of linoleic acid. Some prostaglandin metabolites influence salt and water excretion and can cause contraction or dilation of small blood vessels, thereby affecting blood pressure [50].

4. Cholesterol *gallstones*, precipitated from supersaturated bile, are associated with excess intake of energy and dietary fat [52].

5. A 36-year study on the effect of dietary fat on the progression of *multiple sclerosis* indicated that, with few exceptions, multiple sclerosis patients were very sensitive to or intolerant of saturated fatty acids and that a high animal fat intake might be an important factor in the mechanism of this disease [53].

Digestible Carbohydrates

Functions and Effects of Low Intakes

The primary function of dietary starches and sugars is to provide energy. Fat metabolism in the absence of carbohydrate results in metabolic acidosis due to the buildup of acid end products of fat catabolism. A minimum of 100 g per day of digestible carbohydrate is needed for normal fat metabolism.

Starches and Sugars: Effects of High Intakes

Guidelines from the National Academy of Sciences [5] suggest that 55% or more of the daily energy intake be in the form of carbohydrate that is derived from grain products, legumes, vegetables, and fruit rather than from foods or beverages high in sugars. The US diet derives about 47%–48% of energy from starches and sugars [1]. Sugar intake is estimated to be 62–143 g/day, accounting for 18%–32% of energy intake [54].

Diets containing 60%–70% of calories from starch, such as those consumed in Asian countries, are associated with low plasma cholesterol levels and a low risk for CHD [55]. Intake of starch has been negatively related to CHD, and the effect of starch did not appear to be an indirect effect of lowered fat intake [56]. A review of epidemiologic studies of diet and CHD risk has failed to identify an association with sucrose intake [54]. Recommended treatment for patients with elevated plasma triglyceride and VLDL levels includes weight control, alcohol restriction, increased physical activity, restriction of saturated fat and cholesterol and substitution of carbohydrate for fat. Hypertriglyceridemia can be induced with high-starch (70% of calories) diets, but the effect is temporary and appears to occur mainly after changing from a high-fat to a high-carbohydrate diet [57,58].

Sucrose and fructose have been shown experimentally to promote hypertriglyceridemia in susceptible (carbohydrate-sensitive) individuals. Men appear to be more susceptible than premenopausal women, older persons more than younger persons, and hypertriglyceridemic persons more than normal triglyceridemic persons [59,60].

In experimental animals, meals of relatively high carbohydrate proportions tend to increase brain levels of tryptophan and serotonin [22]. Serotonin-responsive neurons participate in the onset and maintenance of sleep, and the results of a few behavioral tests indicate that meals with a high ratio of carbohydrate to protein increase sleepiness [61].

Epidemiological studies indicate an association between sugar intake and tooth decay [62] and increasing rates of tooth decay among populations whose sugar intake is increasing [63]. Sucrose is converted by mouth bacteria into plaque (extracellular polymers of glucose or fructose), which adheres firmly to tooth surfaces [64]. Bacteria in the plaque readily convert sugars into acids which demineralize teeth. The frequency of sugar consumption and the form in which it is consumed are of concern with regard to tooth decay. Foods that adhere to the teeth are more cariogenic than those that wash off quickly [65]. Also of concern with respect to dental caries are genetics and oral hygiene.

Sugars: Problems

An insufficiency of lactase, the enzyme responsible for the breakdown of lactose (milk sugar) in the small intestine, can cause lactose intolerance, which is characterized by abdominal discomfort, pain, and diarrhea as a result of bacterial action on undigested lactose in the colon. This disorder is most common in Asians, Africans, American Indians and American blacks [66]. Many lactase-deficient individuals can consume modest amounts of lactose-containing foods. They may also consume milk and milk products modified by addition of lactase, and fermented products such as cheese or yogurt.

The inability to convert galactose into glucose because of enzyme deficiencies results in galactosemia. With this disorder, galactose and galactitol increase in the blood and in tissues resulting in liver dysfunction (hepatomegaly and ascites), cataracts, and mental retardation. Galactose, as a constituent of lactose, is found in mammalian milks, milk products, and foods made with milk products. These foods and products containing added lactose (such as medications with lactose filler) must be excluded from the diet. Some fruits, vegetables, and legumes contain galactose, but the amounts are small. If necessary, these foods may also be removed from the diet.

Dietary Fiber

Functions and Effects of Inadequate Intake

Dietary fiber consists of the components of plant materials that resist the action of digestive enzymes and includes cellulose, hemicellulose, lignin, gums, pectins, mucilages and algal polysaccharides. Major food sources of fiber are vegetables, legumes, fruits, and whole grain products. Dietary fiber increases saliva flow, increases satiety, delays digestion and absorption, binds intestinal bile acids, increases the mass of intestinal bacteria, decreases stool transit time, and increases stool weights and frequency of elimination [67]; however, the dietary fibers from different foods have somewhat different effects. The suggested intake for dietary fibers is 20–30 g/day, not to exceed 35 g/day [68]. US intakes average 12 g per day for women and 18 g per day for men [1]. Inadequate intake of dietary fiber can have a number of effects.

1. Inadequate consumption of dietary fiber may result in *constipation*. Increased intake of wheat bran and other sources of dietary fiber prevents constipation and relieves its symptoms [69].

2. *Diverticulitis*, which occurs when diverticula (abnormal outpocketings of the intestinal wall) become infected, results in constipation, diarrhea, flatulence, abdominal pain, fever, and mucus and blood in the stools [70]. Measurements of intestinal transit times, bowel motility, stool weights, and intraluminal pressures [71,72] and international comparisons of fiber intake and disease prevalence rates [73] support the notion that diverticular disease might result from inadequate intake of dietary fiber. Dietary intervention trials have reported beneficial effects of bran and other fiber sources on pain, constipation, and other symptoms as well as on intraluminal pressures [69,72]. Fiber supplements are often used successfully in clinical management of uncomplicated diverticular disease [69].

3. Low-fiber diets ares associated with *gallstone* formation [4]. Cholesterol, precipitated from bile, is the principal component of most gallstones [4]. The binding of cholesterol with fiber in the intestine may stimulate the liver to increase production of bile acids and increase cholesterol solubility [74]. Large doses of wheat bran increase bile cholesterol solubility [75].

4. Water-soluble fiber fractions (e.g., pectin and guar), found in oat bran, guar gum, psyllium seeds, and certain beans, have been shown to have *hypocholesterolemic effects* [76–78]. Addition of fiber to high-carbohydrate diets has been reported to prevent triglyceride elevation that may occur with high-carbohydrate diets [79].

5. Epidemiologic comparisons have associated low-fiber diets with increased prevalence of *appendicitis* [80,81]. It has been reported that children whose fiber intake is in the upper fiftieth percentile have a 50% lower risk of appendicitis [82]. Trends in fiber intake are not, however, consistent with the decline in appendicitis rates during the past few decades, and not all studies have shown that patients with appendicitis consume less fiber than control subjects [83].

6. Dietary fiber may offer a protective effect against *colon cancer* [84–86]. Of 24 correlation studies summarized in the Surgeon General's Report on Nutrition [4], 21 identified an inverse association of dietary fiber, fiber-rich diets, or other measures of fiber consumption with occurrence of colon cancer; three showed no association; and none reported a positive association. The Surgeon General's Report [4] has summarized 19 case-control studies on the role of fiber-containing foods in colon cancer. Three of these studies found no effect, three found an increased risk and 13 observed a protective effect of fiber-containing foods, especially vegetables.

Fiber may exert its protective action in colon cancer by reducing transit time in the bowel and therefore decreasing the time for exposure to potential carcinogens; diluting the concentration of carcinogens in the colon; affecting the production of bile acids and other potential carcinogens in the stool; altering the nature of fecal bile acids by virtue of its influence on the composition and metabolic activity of fecal flora; and/or reducing colonic pH by increasing fermentation and short-chain fatty acid production [87,88].

Effects of Excess

Potential adverse effects of excess dietary fiber include intestinal obstruction (primarily due to gel-forming fiber); interference with absorption of calcium, magnesium, zinc, manganese and iron; inflammation of the bowel mucosa (with certain gums); and colonic volvulus [89]. The most frequently suggested adverse effect of high fiber intake is mineral imbalance; however, consumption of diets containing about 20–25 g of insoluble fiber (30–35 g total dietary fiber) from foods per day does not appear to pose a problem relative to mineral availability [69].

Alcohol

US Intake

Alcohol accounts for 3%–7% of the energy intake of those over 14 years in the US [90]. For drinkers only, alcohol contributes about 10% of the daily energy intake [90]. The drinking profile of the US population has been described as follows:

33% do not drink;
34% are light drinkers (1–3 drinks per week);

24% are moderate drinkers (less than 2 drinks per day); and

9% are heavy drinkers (2 or more drinks per day) [91]

The Surgeon General recommends that if alcohol is used, it should be taken only in moderation (i.e., less than two drinks per day) and that it should not be used during pregnancy or while driving, operating machinery, taking medication, or engaging in activities requiring judgment [4].

Effects of Excess

Alcohol is an addictive drug which can have adverse effects on body cells and tissues. In addition, alcohol can adversely affect behavior, judgment and co-ordination and can result in bodily/emotional harm to others by causing violence and accidents, especially automobile accidents. Alcohol causes injury to organs by direct toxic action (of alcohol or its metabolic by-products) and/or by affecting nutritional status. There seem to be genetic differences in predisposition to the direct toxic effects of alcohol.

1. The consumption of alcohol can diminish nutritional status by reducing intake of essential nutrients, impairing digestion and absorption of nutrients, altering the ability to convert nutrients into active coenzyme forms, and/or increasing excretion of nutrients (e.g., folate, magnesium, calcium and zinc) in the urine. Socioeconomic factors are important with regard to the nutritional status of alcoholics; indigent alcoholics are more malnourished than middle- or upper-class alcoholics [4]. Thiamin and folate deficiencies are the most common nutrient deficiencies associated with alcoholism.

2. Alcohol produces a direct toxic effect on the liver, causing *cirrhosis* in about 12%–15% of alcoholics [4]. Alcoholic hepatitis (alcohol-induced liver inflammation) may respond to improvement in nutritional status (e.g., parenteral infusions of amino acids) [92]. Fatty liver from alcohol consumption results from reduced hepatic oxidation of fatty acids (due to oxidation of alcohol), increased conversion of fatty acids into long-chain fatty acids and triglycerides, and mobilization of fatty acids from muscle and adipose tissue to the liver [4].

3. In alcoholics, *Wernicke–Korsakoff's syndrome*, characterized by weakness of eye movements, gait disturbances, confusion, memory loss, and a disordered sense of time, is caused more by thiamin deficiency than by the direct toxic effect of alcohol [4].

4. Alcoholic *peripheral neuropathy*, results in degeneration of nerve axons that affect the lower extremities [4]. It is a common neurologic complication of alcoholism occurring in over 80% of persons with severe neurologic problems such as Wernicke's encephalopathy [93]. Recovery from alcoholic peripheral neuropathy is slow and often incomplete [4]. Supplementation with B-complex vitamins offers some relief, but abstinence from alcohol is essential for improvement [4].

5. Cerebral atrophy caused by alcohol consumption may be reversed with the cessation of excessive drinking [94], but the associated cognitive dysfunction

(*alcoholic dementia*) is due to a combination of thiamin deficiency and the direct toxic effects of alcohol on the brain [95].

6. Individuals with unexplained acute atrial fibrillation have been shown to have a significantly higher rate of heavy alcohol consumption than control persons [96]. Alcoholics with evidence of myocardial dysfunction are more sensitive to the depressant effects of alcohol on the heart and to atrial and ventricular dysrhythmias after acute administration of alcohol [4].

7. Alcoholic *cardiomyopathy* is caused by the direct toxic effect of alcohol on the myocardium [4]. The changes in the myocardial cells with alcoholic cardiomyopathy are similar to those in the livers of persons with alcoholic liver disease, and the only factor shown significantly to affect recovery is abstinence from alcohol [97]. Acetaldehyde, the first product of alcohol oxidation, may induce the myocardial damage [98]. Acute alcohol ingestion produces dilation of peripheral blood vessels and diminished blood return to the heart and has a depressant effect on heart muscle action [99]. Chronic alcohol use injures the heart muscle, depresses ventricular function, and impairs cardiac performance [4]. Over time, alcohol abuse may lead to irreversible damage to the heart muscle and cause congestive heart failure or cardiac arrhythmias [4].

8. Individuals who regularly consume large amounts of alcohol have higher *blood pressure* than people who abstain from alcohol or who drink only moderate amounts [100]. Consumption of three to four alcoholic drinks per day causes a measurable increase in both the systolic and diastolic blood pressures [4]. As much as 11% of hypertension in men may be attributable to consumption of alcohol [101]. In most US studies, a "J"-shaped association is observed between blood pressure and alcohol consumption, with blood pressure greater in nondrinkers than in those consuming one to two drinks per day [4].

9. The most common lipid abnormality associated with alcohol abuse and alcoholism is *hypertriglyceridemia* with high VLDL levels (type IV hyperlipidemia) [4]. In more severely affected individuals, there may be an accompanying elevation of chylomicrons (type V hyperlipidemia) [4]. Persons with alcohol-induced hyperlipidemia do not respond to dietary or drug intervention unless alcohol intake is limited [102].

10. High alcohol intake has been associated with *CHD* deaths; however, several population studies have suggested that light to moderate drinkers have a lower risk for coronary artery disease than do nondrinkers [103,104]. In alcoholics, the reports to date regarding HDL cholesterol levels have been variable and appear to depend on a variety of factors such as level of alcohol intake, the degree of hepatic microsomal enzyme induction, and the severity of alcoholic liver disease [105]. The epidemiologic findings await further confirmation as well as elucidation of a biologic mechanism to explain the apparent protective effect of alcohol [4].

11. Excessive alcohol intake is a risk factor for *osteoporosis*. In women, the incidence of hip fractures has been observed to increase with increasing alcohol consumption [105]. Bone loss, decreased bone density, increased bone resorp-

tion, and increased fracture incidence have been reported among alcoholics [107,108]. Alcohol-induced bone loss may involve poor nutrition, alcohol-induced calcium diuresis, secondary effects of liver disease, calcium malabsorption, and induction of excessive parathyroid hormone secretion [4].

12. Alcohol-induced *impaired glucose tolerance* and alcohol-induced *hypoglycemia* are of special concern in patients with diabetes mellitus [4]. Associated dietary intake, the level and history of alcohol consumption, and the presence of organ pathology such as hepatic insufficiency are responsible for the wide variation in the effect of alcohol on glucose tolerance [4]. Hypoglycemia may occur with acute alcohol ingestion after minimal food intake for several days or more [4]. Victims have been found stuporous or deeply comatose [4]. Alcohol may block gluconeogenesis, and in the absence of glycogen stores, hypoglycemia may occur. Malnutrition, adrenocortical insufficiency, thyrotoxicosis, and consumption of diets high in protein and low in carbohydrate increase sensitivity to the hypoglycemic effects of alcohol ingestion [4].

13. *Fetal alcohol syndrome* is characterized by facial malformation, prenatal and postnatal growth deficiencies, and central nervous system disorders, including mental retardation [4]. Abnormalities increase in proportion to the dose of alcohol [109,110]. Fetal alcohol syndrome occurs in disproportionately large numbers of American Indians, in patients of lower socioeconomic background, and in children of older mothers, groups among whom the rate of alcohol abuse and alcoholism are higher [111]. The syndrome is due to toxic effects of alcohol and not to nutritional deficiencies [4]. One or two alcoholic drinks per day are associated with higher rates of spontaneous abortion, premature detachment of the placenta, and low birth weight [112,113]. Complete abstinence at the time of conception and during pregnancy is recommended; routine health and prenatal care should include counseling about the hazards of alcohol use [4].

Energy

Effects of Deficiency

Suggested energy intakes for adult women and men in the US are 2000 and 2700 kilocalories per day, respectively [2]; average intakes are 82% and 94%, respectively, of these values [1]. Adequate energy is essential for normal growth and body functioning and is provided by the macronutrients protein, fat, digestible carbohydrate and alcohol. Inadequate energy intake leads to impaired growth, impaired body maintenance, low body fat reserves, wasting of body tissue, symptoms of protein deficiency (as body/dietary protein is burned for fuel) and osteoporosis. Irreparable damage may eventually be done to body organs and tissues (e.g. eyes, bone, kidneys, heart) due to inadequate energy intake.

1. The onset and continuation of menses may depend on a certain body weight or level of fat stores [4]. Healthy women who lose large amounts of weight (e.g. with anorexia nervosa) often stop menstruating.

2. The combination of decreased intake of calories, calcium and other nutrients and decreased production of estrogen may be responsible for reduced density of bone mass in persons with anorexia nervosa [114]. Female athletes, particularly runners and ballet dancers, who have very low body fat content, a low intake of calories and calcium and amenorrhea, also have decreased bone mass [115,116]. Low body fat may also cause reduced bone mass in postmenopausal women [117]. Physical exercise may increase the peak bone mass achieved at maturity and may also reduce losses of bone mass after maturity [118]. Three to four hours of weight-bearing exercise per week are potentially beneficial to the skeleton and could represent a safe, low-cost method for maintaining bone mass [4].

Effects of Excess

1. Excessive energy intake (excessive compared to body requirement) leads to accumulation of body fat (obesity). Obesity is associated with CHD, hypertension, low levels of HDL, elevated plasma glucose levels, high blood cholesterol, elevated LDL, hypertriglyceridemia, diabetes mellitus, and several types of cancer [4]. Obesity is a significant independent predictor of CHD, especially in women and in persons under age 50 [118]. Weight gained in adulthood conveys an added risk [4]. Leanness and avoidance of weight gain before middle age are advisable goals in the prevention of CHD for most men and women [119].

2. The association between body weight and blood pressure has been confirmed [120,121], and elevated blood pressure may be significantly reduced with weight loss [4,100] even in the absence of sodium restriction [122,123]. Control of obesity could eliminate hypertension in 48% of whites and 28% of blacks [124]. Even if weight loss does not reduce blood pressure to normal levels, health risks may be reduced, and smaller doses of antihypertensive medication may be needed [4].

3. Positive associations between increased body weight or increased energy intake and an increased risk for cancer have been observed for cancers of the breast, colon, prostate, endometrium, kidney, cervix and thyroid [4]. Cancer mortality ratios of people who are more than 40% overweight are higher than those of people of average weight by 33% for men and 55% for women [125]. In men, this relationship was statistically significant for cancer of the colon, rectum, and prostate and in women, for cancer of the breast, uterus (cervix and endometrium), ovary and gallbladder. Additional studies are needed to separate the individual effect of energy, fat, and obesity on cancer [126].

4. Cholesterol gallstones are associated with obesity [127] and with excess intake of energy and fat [52].

Summary

This chapter has reviewed the effects of deficient and excessive intakes of energy and of the macronutrients protein, fat, digestible carbohydrates, dietary fiber, and alcohol. Nutritional concerns regarding these substances vary within and among countries, depending on the types and amounts of foods that are available and the economic resources of the people. Desirable daily intakes for energy and macronutrients for various age-sex groups are generally known, but it is difficult to determine at what levels problems of deficiency and excess occur. Problem levels depend on individual tolerances and are in part determined by genetics, age, sex, body size and build, level of physical activity, environmental factors, and previous exposures. Also of concern are inborn errors of metabolism and other disorders or diseases that may affect the body's ability to utilize specific macronutrients. Assessments of the relationship of energy and the macro-nutrients to health require continuation of current studies with greater refine-ment and precision. Sources of error that lead to inconclusive and/or conflicting results might be eliminated by improving techniques of assessing what people eat and the quantities consumed; improving estimates of macronutrient intakes as derived from food consumption data (i.e., improvement in food composition databases); refining the physiological, biochemical and clinical markers that are related to macronutrient status; and assuring that studies are properly designed and controlled.

Acknowledgments. The Surgeon General's Report on Nutrition and Health [4] and the National Academy of Sciences' Report on Diet and Health [5] are the most recent, comprehensive, and authoritative reviews of the scientific literature concerning the relationship of diet to health and disease. Information from these two sources concerning macronutrients has been abstracted for this chapter.

References

1. Human Nutrition Information Service (1985/1986) CSFII. Nationwide Food Con-sumption Survey. Continuing Survey of Food Intakes by Individuals. Women 19–50 years and their children 1–5 years, 1 day 1985 (report no. 85-1, Nov. 1985). Men 19–50 years, 1 day (report no. 85-3, Nov. 1986). US Department of Agriculture, Washington, DC
2. Committee on Dietary Allowances, Food and Nutrition Board, National Research Council (1980) Recommended Dietary Allowances. 9th rev ed., National Academy of Sciences, Washington, DC
3. US Dept of Agriculture and US Dept of Health and Human Services (1985) Nutrition and your health. Dietary guidelines for Americans. 2nd ed. Home and Garden Bulle-tin No. 232. Washington, DC
4. US Dept of Health and Human Services, Public Health Service (1988) The Surgeon General's report on nutrition and health. DHHS publication no. (PHS) 88-50210. Superintendent of Documents, U.S. Government Printing Office, Washington DC
5. Committee on Diet and Health, Food and Nutrition Board, National Academy of Sciences (1989) Diet and health: implications for reducing chronic disease risk. National Academy Press, Washington, DC
6. West RO, Hayes OB (1968) Diet and serum cholesterol levels. A comparison between vegetarians and nonvegetarians in a Seventh-Day Adventist group. Am J Clin Nutr 21:853–862

7. Descovitch GC, Ceredi C, Gaddi A et al. (1980) Multicentre study of soybean protein diet for outpatient hypercholesterolemic patients. Lancet ii:709–712
8. Sirtori CR, Gatti E, Mantero O (1979) Clinical experience with soybean protein diet in the treatment of hypercholesterolemia. Am J Clin Nutr 21:853–862
9. Armstrong B, Doll R (1975) Environmental factors and cancer incidence and mortality in different countries, with special reference to dietary practices. Int J Cancer 15:617–631
10. Kolonel LN (1987) Fat and colon cancer: how firm is the evidence? Am J Clin Nutr 45:336–341
11. Lubin JH, Wax Y, Modan B (1986) Role of fat, animal protein, and dietary fiber in breast cancer etiology: a case-control study. J Natl Cancer Inst 77:605–611
12. Jain M, Cook GM, Davis FG, Grace MG, Howe GR, Miller AB (1980) A case-control study of diet and colo-rectal cancer. Int J Cancer 26:757–768
13. Potter JD, McMichael AJ (1986) Diet and cancer of the colon and rectum: a case-control study. J Natl Cancer Inst 76:557–569
14. Lubin JH, Burns PE, Blot WJ, Ziegler RG, Lees AW, Fraumeni JF (1981) Dietary factors and breast cancer risk. Int J Cancer 28:685–689
15. Haenszel W, Berg JW, Segi M, Kurihara M, Locke FB (1973) Large-bowel cancer in Hawaiian Japanese. J Natl Cancer Inst 51:1765–1779
16. Heaney RP, Gallagher JC, Johnston CC, Neer R, Parfitt AM, Whedon GD. Calcium nutrition and bone health in the elderly. Am J Clin Nutr 36:986–1013
17. Hegsted DM (1986) Calcium and osteoporosis. J Nutr 116:2316–2319
18. Hostetter TH, Olson JL, Rennke HG, Venkatachalam MA, Brenner BM (1981) Hyperfiltration in remnant nephrons: a potentially adverse response to renal ablation. Am J Physiol 241:F85–93
19. Brenner BM, Meyer TW, Hostetter TH (1982) Dietary protein intake and the progressive nature of kidney disease: the role of hemodynamically mediated glomerular injury in the pathogenesis of progressive glomerular sclerosis in aging, renal ablation, and intrinsic renal disease. N Engl J Med 307:652–659
20. Hartmann E (1982) Effects of L-tryptophan on sleepiness and on sleep. In: Leiberman HR, Wurtman RJ (eds) Research strategies for assessing the behavioral effects of foods and nutrients. Center for Brain Sciences and Metabolism, Cambridge, MA, pp 12–29
21. Jenicke M (1985) Drug treatment of insomnia. Top Geriatr 3:29–32
22. Wurtman RJ, Hefti H, Melamed E (1981) Precursor control of neurotransmitter synthesis. Pharmacol Rev 32:315–335
23. Hosobuchi Y, Lamb S, Bascom D (1980) Tryptophan loading may reverse tolerance to opiate analgesics in humans: a preliminary report. Pain 9:161–169
24. King RB (1980) Pain and tryptophan. J Neurosurg 53:44–52
25. Growdon JH, Melamed E (1982) Effects of oral L-tyrosine administration on CSF tyrosine and homovanillic acid levels in patients with Parkinson's disease. Life Sci 30:827–832
26. Growdon JH (1981) Tyrosine treatment in Parkinson's disease: clinical effects. Neurology 31:143
27. Van Praag HM, Lemus C (1986) Monoamine precursors in the treatment of psychiatric disorder. In: Wurtman RJ, Wurtman JJ (eds) Nutrition and the brain, vol 7. Raven, New York, pp 89–138
28. Leonard CD, Luke RG, Siegel RR (1975) Parenteral essential amino acids in acute renal failure. Urology VI:154–157

29. Feinstein EI, Blumenkrantz MJ, Healy M et al. (1981) Clinical and metabolic responses to parenteral nutrition in acute renal failure – a controlled double-blind study. Medicine (Baltimore) 60:124–137

30. Feinstein EI, Kopple JD, Silberman H et al. (1983) Total parenteral nutrition with high or low nitrogen intake in patients with acute renal failure. Kidney Int 24 (suppl 16):S319–323

31. Chandra RK (1981) Immunodeficiency in undernutrition and overnutrition. Nutr Rev 39:225–231

32. Hornstra G (1980) Dietary prevention of coronary heart disease. Effect of dietary fats on arterial thrombosis. Postgrad Med J 56:563–570

33. Renaud S (1987) Nutrients, platelet functions and coronary heart disease. In: Somoygi JC, Renaud S, Astier-Dumas M (eds) Emerging problems in human nutrition, bibliotheca nutritio et Dieta, vol 40. Karger, Basel, pp 1–17

34. Hornstra G, Chait A, Karvonen MJ, Lewis B, Turpeinen O, Vergroesen AJ (1973) Influence of dietary fat on platelet function in men. Lancet i:1155–1157

35. Jakubowski JA, Ardlie NG (1978) Modification of human platelet function in a diet enriched in saturated or polyunsaturated fat. Atherosclerosis 31:335–344

36. Kromhout D, Bosschieter EB, Coulander CL (1985) The inverse relation between fish consumption and 20 year mortality from coronary heart disease. N Engl J Med 312:1205–1224

37. Dyerberg J, Jorgensen KA (1982) Marine oils and thrombogenesis. Progn Lipid Res 21:225–269

38. Fehily AM, Burr ML, Phillips KM, Deadman NM (1983) The effect of fatty fish on plasma lipid and lipoprotein concentrations. Am J Clin Nutr 38:349–351

39. von Lossonczy TO, Ruiter A, Bronsegeest-Schoute HC, van Gent CM, Hermus RJJ (1978) The effect of a fish diet on serum lipids in healthy human subjects. Am J Clin Nutr 31:1340–1346

40. Saynor R, Verel D, Gillott J (1984) The long-term effect of dietary supplementation with fish lipid concentrate on serum lipids, bleeding time, platelets, and angina. Atherosclerosis 50:3–10

41. Harris WS, Connor WE (1980) The effects of salmon oil upon plasma lipids, lipoprotein, and triglyceride clearance. Trans Assoc Am Physicians 93:148–155

42. Nestel PJ, Connor WE, Reardon MF, Connor S, Wong S, Boston R (1984) Suppression by diets rich in fish oil of very low density lipoprotein production in man. J Clin Invest 74:82–89

43. Wynder EL, McCoy GD, Reddy BS et al. (1981) Nutrition and metabolic epidemiology of cancers of the oral cavity, esophagus, colon, breast, prostate and stomach. In: Newell GR, Ellison NM (eds) Nutrition and cancer: etiology and treatment. Raven, New York, pp 11–48

44. Rose DP (1986) The biochemical epidemiology of prostatic carcinoma. In: Ip C, Birt DF, Rogers AE, Mettlin C (eds) Dietary fat and cancer. Liss, New York, pp 43–68

45. Rose DP, Boyar AP, Wynder EL (1986) International comparisons of mortality rates for cancer of the breast, ovary, prostate, and colon, and per capita food consumption. Cancer 58:2363–2371

46. Mahboubi E, Eyler N, Wynder EL (1982) Epidemiology of cancer of the endometrium. Clin Obstet Gynecol 25:5–17

47. Carroll KK, Khor HT (1975) Dietary fat in relation to tumorigenesis. Prog Biochem Pharmacol 10:308–353

48. Iacono JM, Puska P, Dougherty RM. (1983) Effect of dietary fat on blood pressure in a rural Finnish population. Am J Clin Nutr 38:860–869

49. Puska P, Iacono JM, Nissinen A et al. (1985) Dietary fat and blood pressure: an intervention study on the effects of a low-fat diet with two levels of polyunsaturated fat. Prev Med 14:573–584

50. Iacono JM, Judd JT, Marshall MW et al. (1981) The role of dietary essential fatty acids and prostaglandins in reducing blood pressure. Prog Lipid Res 20:349–364

51. Iacono JM, Dougherty RM, Puska P (1982) Reduction of blood pressure associated with dietary polyunsaturated fat. Hypertension 4:34–42

52. Heaton K (1985) Gallstones. In: Trowell H, Burkitt D, Heaton K (eds) Dietary fibre, fibre-depleted foods and disease. Academic Press, New York, pp 289–304

53. Swank RL, Grimsgaard A (1988) Multiple sclerosis: the lipid relationship. Am J Clin Nutr 48:1387–1393

54. Glinsmann WH, Irausquin H, Park YK (1986) Evaluation of health aspects of sugar contained in carbohydrate sweeteners: report of Sugars Task Force. J Nutr 116(11S): S1–S216

55. Keys A (ed) (1970) Coronary heart disease in seven countries. Circulation 41 (suppl 1)

56. Gordon T, Kagan A, Garcia-Palmieri MR et al. (1981) Diet and its relation to coronary heart disease and death in three populations. Circulation 63:500–515

57. Little JA, McGuire V, Derksen A (1979) Available carbohydrates. In: Levy R, Rifkind B, Dennis B, Ernst N (eds) Nutrition, lipids, and coronary heart disease. Raven, New York, pp 119–148

58. Ahrens EH (1986) Carbohydrates, plasma triglycerides, and coronary heart disease. Nutr Rev 44:60–64

59. Reiser S, Bickard MC, Hallfrisch J, Michaelis IV OE, Prather ES (1981) Blood lipids and their distribution in lipoproteins in hyperinsulinemic subjects fed three different levels of sucrose. J Nutr 111:1045–1057

60. Coulston AM, Hollenback CB, Swislocki ALM, Chen YDI, Raven GM (1987) Deleterious metabolic effects of high-carbohydrate sucrose-containing diets in patients with non-insulin-dependent diabetes mellitus. Am J Med 82:213–220

61. Lieberman HR, Spring B, Garfield GS (1986) The behavioral effects of food constituents: strategies used in studies of amino acids, protein, carbohydrate and caffeine. Nutr Rev 44 (May Suppl):61–70

62. Sreebny LM (1982) Sugar availability, sugar consumption and dental caries. Community Dent Oral Epidemiol 10:1–7

63. Burt BA, Ismail AI (1986) Diet, nutrition and cariogenicity. J Dent Res 65 (spec iss):1475–1484

64. Gibbons RJ, van Houte J (1978) Cariology. Section B: Bacteriology of dental caries. In: Shaw JH, Sweeney EA, Cappuccino CC, Meller SM (eds) Textbook of oral biology. Saunders, Philadelphia, pp 975–991

65. Gustafsson BE, Quensel CE, Lanke LS et al. (1954) The Vipeholm dental caries study: the effect of different levels of carbohydrate intake on caries activity in 436 individuals observed for five years. Acta Odontol Scand 11:232–364

66. Gray GM (1983) Intestinal disaccharidase deficiencies and glucose-galactose malabsorption. In: Stanbury JB, Wyngaarden JB, Frederickson DS (eds) The metabolic basis of inherited disease. 5th edn, McGraw-Hill, New York, pp 1729–1742

67. Trowell H, Burkitt D, Heaton K (1985) Definitions of dietary fibre and fibre-depleted foods. In: Trowell H, Burkitt D, Heaton K (eds) Dietary fibre, fibre-depleted foods and disease. Academic Press, New York, pp 21–30

68. Butrum RR, Clifford CK, Lanza E (1988) NCI dietary guidelines: rationale. Am J Clin Nutr 48 (suppl)
69. Pilch SM (ed) (1987) Life Science Research Office. Physiological effects and health consequences of dietary fiber. FASEB, Bethesda, MD
70. Almy TP, Howell DA (1980) Diverticular disease of the colon. N Engl J Med 302:324–331
71. Burkitt DP, Walker ARP, Painter NS (1974) Dietary fiber and disease. JAMA 229:1068–1074
72. Painter N (1985) Diverticular disease of the colon. In: Trowell H, Burkitt D, Heaton K (eds) Dietary fibre, fibre-depleted foods and disease. Academic Press, New York, pp 145–160
73. Mendeloff AI (1986) Thoughts on the epidemiology of diverticular disease. Baillieres Clin Gastroenterol 15:855–877
74. Strasberg SM, Petrunka CN, Ilson RG (1976) Effect of bile acid synthesis rate on cholesterol secretion rate in the steady state. Gastroenterology 71:1067–1070
75. Pomare EW, Heaton KW, Low-Beer TS, Espiner HJ (1976) The effect of wheat bran upon bile salt metabolism and upon the lipid composition of bile in gallstone patients. Am J Dig Dis 21:521–526
76. Jenkins DJA, Leeds AR, Newton C, Cummings JH (1975) Effect of pectin, guar gum and wheat fiber on serum cholesterol. Lancet i:1116–1117
77. Kirby RW, Anderson JW, Sieling B et al. (1981) Oat-bran intake selectively lowers serum low-density lipoprotein cholesterol concentrations of hypercholesterolemic men. Am J Clin Nutr 34:824–829
78. Anderson JW, Story L, Sieling B, Chen WJL, Petro MS, Story J (1984) Hypocholesterolemic effects of oat-bran or bean intake for hypercholesterolemic men. Am J Clin Nutr 40:1146–1155
79. Anderson JW, Chen WL, Sieling B (1980) Hypolipidemic effects of high-carbohydrate, high fiber diets. Metabolism 29:551–558
80. Segal I (1985) Hiatal hernia and gastroesophageal reflux. In: Trowell H, Burkitt D, Heaton K (eds) Dietary fibre, fibre-depleted foods and disease. Academic Press, New York, pp 241–248
81. Walker A, Burkitt D (1985) Appendicitis. In: Trowell H, Burkitt D, Heaton K (eds) Dietary fibre, fibre-depleted foods and disease. Academic Press, New York, pp 191–203
82. Brender JD, Weiss NS, Koepsell TD, Marcuse EK (1985) Fiber intake and childhood appendicitis. Am J Public Health 75:399–400
83. Cove-Smith JR, Langman MJS (1975) Appendicitis and dietary fibre. Gut 16:409
84. Burkitt DP (1980) Fiber in the etiology of colorectal cancer. In: Winawer SJ, Schottenfeld D, Sherlock P (eds) Progress in cancer research and therapy, vol 13. Raven, New York, pp 13–18
85. Reddy BS (1982) Dietary fiber and colon carcinogenesis: a critical review. In: Vahouny GV, Kritchevsky D (eds) Dietary fiber in health and disease. Plenum, New York, pp 265–285
86. Greenwald P, Lanza E, Eddy GA (1987) Dietary fiber in the reduction of colon cancer risk. J Am Diet Assoc 87:1178–1188
87. Committee on Diet, Nutrition, and Cancer, National Research Council, National Academy of Sciences (1982) Diet, nutrition, and cancer. National Academy Press, Washington, DC

88. Eastwood MA, McKay LF, Brydon WG (1986) Methane production and excretion: a marker of cecal fermentation. In: Vahouny GV, Kritchevsky D (eds) Dietary fiber: basic and clinical aspects. Plenum, New York, pp 151–166

89. Klurfeld DM (1987) The role of dietary fiber in gastrointestinal disease. J Am Diet Assoc 87:1172–1176

90. Williamson DF, Forman MR, Binkin NJ, Gentry EM, Remington PL, Trowbridge FL (1987) Alcohol and body weight in United States adults. Am J Public Health 77:1324–1330

91. Moore MH, Gerstein DR (eds) (1981) Alcohol and public policy: beyond the shadow of prohibition. National Academy Press, Washington, DC

92. Nasrallah SM, Galambos JT (1980) Amino acid therapy of alcoholic hepatitis. Lancet ii:1276–1277

93. Victor M, Adams RD, Collins GH (1971) The Wernicke–Korsakoff syndrome. Davis, Philadelphia

94. Ron MA, Acker W, Shaw GK et al. (1982) Computerized tomography of the brain in chronic alcoholism: a survey and follow-up study. Brain 105:497–514

95. Nakada T, Knight RT (1984) Alcohol and the central nervous system. Med Clin North Am 68:121–131

96. Rich EC, Siebold C, Campion B (1985) Alcohol-related acute atrial fibrillation. Arch Intern Med 145:830–833

97. Demakis JG, Proskey A, Rahimtoola SH et al. (1974) The natural course of alcoholic cardiomyopathy. Ann Intern Med 80:293–297

98. Schreiber SS, Briden K, Oratz M, Rothschild MA (1972) Ethanol, acetaldehyde, and myocardial protein synthesis. J Clin Invest 51:2820–2826

99. Lang RM, Borrow KM, Neumann A, Feldman T (1985) Adverse cardiac effects of acute alcohol ingestion in young adults. Ann Intern Med 102:742–747

100. MacMahon SW (1987) Alcohol consumption and hypertension. Hypertension 9:111–121

101. MacMahon SW (1986) Alcohol and hypertension: implications for prevention and treatment (editorial). Ann Intern Med 105:124–126

102. Janus ED, Lewis B (1978) Alcohol and abnormalities of lipid metabolism. Clin Endocrinol Metab 7:321–332

103. Yano K, Rhoads GG, Kagan A (1977) Coffee, alcohol and risk of coronary heart disease among Japanese men living in Hawaii. N Engl J Med 297:405–409

104. Blackwelder WC, Yano K, Rhoads GG, Kagan A, Gordon T, Palesch Y (1980) Alcohol and mortality: the Honolulu Heart Study. Am J Med 68:164–169

105. Hurt RD, Briones ER, Offord KP et al. (1986) Plasma lipids and lipoprotein AI and AII levels in alcoholic patients. Am J Clin Nutr 43:521–529

106. Paganini-Hill A, Ross RK, Gerkins VR, Henderson BE, Arthur M, Mack TM (1981) Menopausal estrogen therapy and hip fractures. Ann Intern Med 95:28–31

107. Nordin BEC (ed) (1984) Metabolic bone and stone disease. Churchill Livingstone, New York

108. Spencer H, Rubio N, Rubio E, Indreika M, Seitam A (1986) Chronic alcoholism: frequently overlooked cause of osteoporosis in men. Am J Med 80:393–397

109. American Medical Association, Council on Scientific Affairs (1983) Fetal effects of maternal alcohol use. JAMA 249:2517–2521

110. Ernhart CB (1987) Alcohol teratogenicity in the human: a detailed assessment of specificity, critical period, and threshold. Am J Obstet Gynecol 156:33–39

111. Streissguth AP (1978) Fetal alcohol syndrome: an epidemiological perspective. Am J Epidemiol 107:467–478

112. Mills JL, Graubard BI, Harley EE, Rhoads GG, Berendes HW (1984) Maternal alcohol consumption and birth weight. JAMA 252:1875–1879

113. Council on Scientific Affairs (1983) Fetal effects on maternal alcohol use. JAMA 249:2517–2521

114. Rigotti NA, Nussbaum SR, Herzog DB, Neer RM (1984) Osteoporosis in women with anorexia nervosa. N Engl J Med 311:1601–1606

115. Drinkwater BL, Nilson K, Chestnut CH, Brenner WJ, Shainholtz S, Southworth MB (1984) Bone mineral content of amenorrheic and eumenorrheic athletes. N Engl J Med 311:277–281

116. Marcus R, Cann C, Madvig P et al. (1985) Menstrual function and bone mass in elite women distance runners: endocrine and metabolic features. Ann Intern Med 102:158–163

117. Dequeker J, Goris P, Uyterhoeven R (1983) Osteoporosis and osteoarthritis (osteoarthrosis). JAMA 249:1448–1451

118. Block JE, Smith R, Black D, Genant HK (1987) Does exercise prevent osteoporosis? JAMA 257:3115–3117

119. Hubert HB, Feinleib M, McNamara PM, Castelli WP (1983) Obesity as an independent risk factor for cardiovascular disease: a 26-year follow-up of participants in the Framingham Heart Study. Circulation 67:968–977

120. Dustan HP (1983) Mechanisms of hypertension associated with obesity. Ann Intern Med 98 (5, suppl, pt 2):860–863

121. Havlik RJ, Hubert HB, Fabsitz R, Feinleib M (1983) Weight and hypertension. Ann Intern Med 98 (5, suppl, pt 2):855–859

122. Reisin E, Abel R, Modan M, Silverberg DS, Eliahou HE, Modan B (1978) Effect of weight loss without salt restriction on the reduction of blood pressure in overweight hypertensive patients. N Engl J Med 298:1–10

123. Maxwell MH, Kushiro T, Dornfeld LP, Tuck ML, Waks AU (1984) Blood pressure changes in obese hypertensive subjects during rapid weight loss: comparison of restricted versus unchanged salt intake. Arch Intern Med 144:1581–1584

124. Tyroler HA, Heyden S, Hames CG (1975) Weight and hypertension: Evans County studies of blacks and whites. In: Paul O (ed) Epidemiology and control of hypertension. Stratton, New York, pp 177–205

125. Garfinkel L (1985) Presentation before the American Cancer Society 2nd National Conference on Diet, Nutrition, and Cancer. Houston, TX

126. Willett WC (1987) Implications of total energy intake for epidemiologic studies of breast and large-bowel cancer. Am J Clin Nutr 45:354–360

127. Diehl AH, Haffner SM, Hazuda HP, Stern MP (1987) Coronary risk factors and clinical gallbladder disease: an approach to the prevention of gallstones? Am J Public Health 77:841–845

CHAPTER 14

The Purchasing Method for the Estimation of Vitamins and Minerals Intake of the Adult

J.P. Mareschi[1]

In industrialized countries, the change in lifestyle, which occurred during the last few decades, and food abundance have brought about a change in eating habits [1]. In the context of this change there can be either an increase or a reduction in energy, but both may involve an inadequate mineral and vitamin intake which may become worse by an increased intake of a more "refined" food. In affluent societies the irrationality of nutritional behavior includes not only the choice of foods, but also the way of preparing and cooking them, the distribution of meals during the day, and some lifestyles that may be connected with the nutritional process. Generally speaking the most frequent errors of the diet, observed in different industrialized countries are as shown in Table 14.1. This trend has been confirmed in France [2,3]. Unfortunately in many countries, including France, there have been only a few surveys of food intake and relative nutritional status; in France most of the available data concern iron.

In order to obtain an overview of the situation in France the "purchasing method" based on data obtained by investigations realized by INSEE [4] has been used. The aims of this chapter are:

1. To explain this method
2. To calculate the intake of vitamins and minerals
3. To discuss its validity comparing results obtained by this method to other ones obtained by surveys on nutrient intake and relative nutritional status
4. To try to define the groups of the population and micronutrients at risk.

Materials and Methods

INSEE (Institut National de la Statistique et des Etudes Economiques) has registered, since 1965, purchases during 8 days, taking as a sample 10000 house-

[1]Directeur des Relations Scientifiques et Administratives, Groupe BSN, 7 rue de Téhéran, F-75381 Paris Cedex 08, France.

Table 14.1. Frequent errors of the diet

| Food intake | | Intake of other components | |
Excess	Deficient	(abuse)	Life habits
Lipids	Cereals[a]	Cigarette smoking	Stress
Alcohol	Vegetables	Oral contraceptive	Sedentary
		Drugs (laxatives, anti- depressive, tranquilizers, etc.)	
Protein (from meat, cheese)	Fruits[b]		
NaCl	Vegetables[b]		
Coffee	Fish		
Sugars	Milk		
	Water		

[a]The cereals often are too refined and it leads to a fibre defect.
[b]The intake of fruits and vegetables is often too low to reach the required value of certain nutrients, such as vitamins, minerals and dietary fibre.

holds from all over France. The results are expressed in quantities per person/ year. The investigation also considers the consumption of home-grown food (vegetables from the kitchen garden), but excludes all the meals taken away from home (canteen, etc.).

From data published by INSEE, a basic daily menu has been established by calculating the quantities per day. The average basic menu provides an energy intake of 2054 kcal/day (proteins: 15.5%, lipids: 44.5% and carbohydrates 40% of the consumed energy), and it does not include the beverages.

The 66 foods or food groups used to start with were later reduced to 55 foods or food groups. This reduction was done by the regrouping the foods similar in composition or in accordance with the frequency of consumption of each. However, for reasons that will be discussed later, the data published by INSEE underestimate the consumption by the adult. Therefore a basic menu has been established from a derived menu corresponding to a more realistic energy intake by an adult. As there is no survey referring to the representative energy intake of the French adult, the recommended energy allowances [5] for men, women, lactating and pregnant women were taken into consideration. Consequently, from a basic menu of 2054 kcal/day derived menus calculations were made of recommended energy allowances for men (2700 kcal/day), women (2000 kcal/day) and pregnant or lactating women (2500 kcal/day). By using this method of calculation the original relationship between the different foods found in the basic menu was retained. Thus the intake of vitamins and minerals was established from the derived menus, with the help of the tables of composition from Souci et al. [6] or, Paul et al. [7].

The calculation was carried out on raw foods for minerals and on cooked foods for vitamins. Vitamins and minerals intake thus calculated do not include those

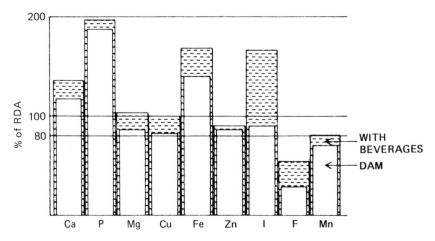

Figure 14.1. Amount of minerals and trace elements supplied by a 2700 kcal daily adjusted menu (DAM) (adult man) (with beverages) [9].

coming from beverages. To estimate the contribution of beverages to the total intake of minerals, another survey [8] was used, because INSEE underestimated the real consumption of beverages. This study shows that minerals, except for calcium and fluoride, are mostly supplied by alcoholic beverages. For this reason only the mineral intake has been considered for men in the estimation of the total mineral food intakes [9] (Fig. 14.1).

With vitamins, no such contribution was taken into consideration as, in general, alcoholic beverages (quantity and quality) are not a major source of vitamins [10]. The data for selenium and chromium were not kept because the values taken from the tables differed too much. Elements with a higher intake than their need were not analyzed (e.g. sodium, potassium). The intake of pantothenic acid is not well known as the gut's ability for biosynthesis of this vitamin is not known and also the analytical method is not reliable. The vitamin niacin intakes are probably underestimated because the niacin equivalent coming from tryptophan ingestion is neglected. On the other hand biotin has not been studied because many data are missing in food composition tables and the contribution of biosynthesis in the gut to the biotin food intake is unknown. Once calculated, vitamins and minerals intake, provided by food, were compared with the recommended dietary allowances for the three types of the considered population.

For vitamin A intake (retinol) the value of vitamin A and other provitamin A products were expressed separately. It was considered advisable to consider that the free retinol intake has to be at least equal to 50% of the recommended total vitamin A intake.

Anderson et al. [11] has established a relationship between the level of mineral intake as compared with the recommended allowances and the probability that

Table 14.2. Minerals intake supplied by a INSEE diet (observed) and percentage of RDA covered by this diet

	Quantity of mineral supplied								
	Ca[a]	P[a]	Mg[a]	Cu[b]	Fe[a]	Zn[a]	I[a]	F[b]	Mn[b]
RDA for women (2000 kcal)	800	800	350	2.5	18	15	0.12	2.7	3.8
RDA for pregnant and lactating women (2500 kcal)	1100	1200	400	2.5	20	22.5	0.14	2.7	3.8
RDA for man (2700 kcal)	800	800	350	2.5	10	15	0.12	2.7	3.8
INSEE (2054 kcal) (Basic daily menu)	726	1168	243	1.6	11.1	10.3	0.08	0.5	2.2
INSEE (2000 kcal)[c]	706	1137	236	1.6	10.8	10	0.08	0.5	2.2
INSEE (2500 kcal)[c]	883	1421	295	2	13.5	12.5	0.1	0.6	2.7
INSEE (2700 kcal)[c]	954	1535	319	2.1	14.6	13.5	0.1	0.7	2.9
	Percentage of RDA								
INSEE 2000/RDA	88	142	67	64	60	67	67	19	58
INSEE 2500/RDA	80	118	74	80	68	56	71	22	71
INSEE 2700/RDA	119	192	91	84	146	90	83	26	76

From: [a]Dupin [5]; [b]Committee on Dietary Allowances [15]
[c]Derived from INSEE 2054 kcal.

the population has an adequate or insufficient supply of minerals. The level of 80% of the recommended allowances appeared to be a critical level below which there is probability of deficiency. For this level of 80%, Anderson showed that there is a 30% probability that the population will receive amounts of minerals below the recommended allowances.

Results

The vitamins and minerals intake supplied by the menus derived from the basic menu, are expressed as percentages of the recommended dietary allowances for men, women and pregnant and lactating women (Tables 14.2 and 14.3; Figs. 14.2–14.7). The elements with a risk of a deficient intake (elements intake lower

Table 14.3. Vitamins intake supplied by a INSEE diet (observed) and percentage of RDA covered by this diet

	Vitamins									
	Total A[a]	Tocopherol[b]	B1	B2	B6	B12	C	PP	AP	AF
RDA for women (2000 kcal)	800	10.06	1.3	1.5	2	0.003	80	15	8.5	0.4
RDA for pregnant and lactating women (2500 kcal)	1300	10.06	1.8	1.8	2.5	0.004	90	20	8.5	0.65
RDA for man (2700 kcal)	1000	10.06	1.5	1.8	2.2	0.003	80	18	8.5	0.4
INSEE (2054 kcal) (Basic daily menu)	1206	7.7	0.89	1.2	1.4	0.005	68	11.2	4.6	0.2
INSEE (2000 kcal)[c]	1180	7.5	0.9	1.2	1.3	0.005	66	11	4.5	0.2
INSEE (2500 kcal)[c]	1470	9.3	1.1	1.4	1.7	0.006	83	14	5.7	0.3
INSEE (2700 kcal)[c]	1593	10.1	1.2	1.6	1.8	0.006	89	15	6.1	0.3
	Percentage of RDA									
INSEE 2000/RDA	148	75	69	80	65	167	83	73	53	50
INSEE 2500/RDA	113	92	61	78	68	150	92	70	67	46
INSEE 2700/RDA	159	100	80	89	82	200	111	83	72	75

From Dupin [5].
[a]Provitamin A represents 68% of total vitamin A in INSEE 2054 kcal, INSEE 2000 kcal and INSEE 2500 kcal and 67% of INSEE 2700 kcal.
[b]Tocopherol is calculated as α-tocopherol equivalents.
[c]Derived from INSEE 2054 kcal.

than 80% of the recommended one) are shown in Table 14.4. The results show that below 2700 kcal/day, it becomes difficult to achieve the recommended dietary allowances with commonly used food.

Discussion

Criticism of the Purchasing Method

The registered purchasing values do not consider consumption away from home. Therefore if "purchasing" is compared with "consumption," the real quantities

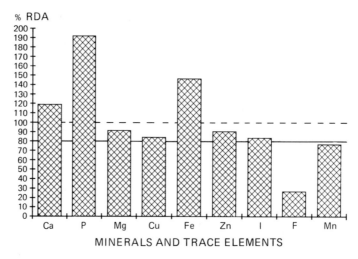

Figure 14.2. Percentage of RDA of minerals and trace elements supplied by 2700 kcal adjusted diet (adult man).

are underestimated. However, the housekeeper cannot consume all she buys in one week, which lessens the error committed in this comparison. Nevertheless, these purchasing values concern all members of a household including children and infants, but children and particularly infants eat much less than adults. This results in an underestimation of intake by an adult which explains the low energy

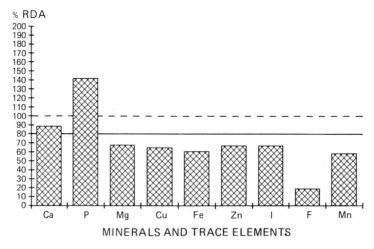

Figure 14.3. Percentage of minerals and trace elements supplied 2000 kcal adjusted diet (adult woman).

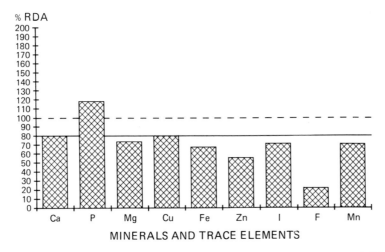

Figure 14.4. Percentage of RDA of minerals and trace elements supplied by a 2500 kcal adjusted diet (pregnant women).

values of the basic menu estimated by INSEE (2054 kcal). These therefore cannot be applied to an adult and menus have to be created (derived) which are closer to the true consumption by an adult, by simply transferring arithmetically the data of the basic menu. The authors of the INSEE survey concluded that the beverage intakes, principally alcoholic beverages, are under-

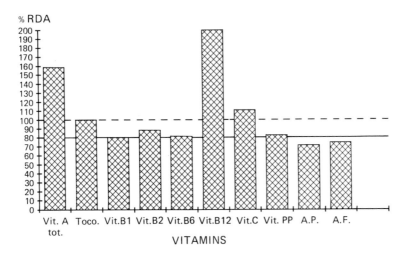

Figure 14.5. Percentage of RDA of vitamins supplied by 2700 kcal adjusted diet (adult man).

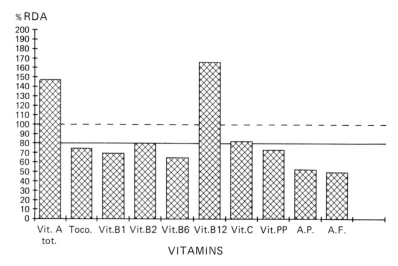

Figure 14.6. Percentage of RDA of vitamins supplied by a 2000 kcal adjusted diet (adult women).

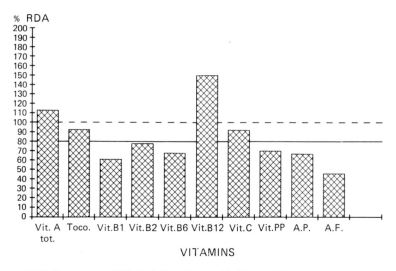

Figure 14.7. Percentage of RDA of vitamins supplied by a 2500 kcal adjusted diet (pregnant women).

Table 14.4. Micronutrients "at risk" in the French adult population diet (INSEE) [13]

	Minerals	Vitamins
Adult man (2700 kcal)	F > Mn	Folic acid > Pantothenic acid > (B1)
Adult woman (2000 kcal)	F > Mn > Fe > Cu > Zn > Mg > I	Folic acid > Panto. acid > B1 > B6 > Toco > (B2)
Pregnant lactating women (2500 kcal)	F > Zn > Fe > Mn > Mg > I > Ca > Cu	Folic acid > B1 > Pantothenic acid > B6 > Free Vit. A

estimated. As already stated, the contribution of beverages to the mineral intake was not taken into account here as it does not greatly change the conclusions of this study.

Validity of the Purchasing Method

This method, even incomplete, shows results very close to those given by other surveys on food intake and surveys on nutritional status, carried out in different industrialized countries (Tables 14.5 and 14.6) [12].

On the other hand, the analysis of the balanced menus (on the basis of energy, proteins, lipids and carbohydrates) leads to slightly higher values for vitamins and minerals, than those given by the purchasing method; the trend of these intakes is nearly the same in both cases [13,14].

Table 14.5. Mineral content of diet: US food survey results (1982–1984) [16]

	Age	Minerals < 80% of RDA or ESADDI[a]
Infant	6–11 months	Cu
Child	2 years	Cu, Fe, Zn
Girl	14–16 years	Cu, Fe, Ca, Mg, Zn, Mn
Boy	14–16 years	Cu, Mg
Woman	25–30 years	Cu, Fe, Mg, Zn, Ca
Man	25–30 years	Cu
Woman	60–65 years	Cu, Zn, Mg, Ca
Man	60–65 years	Cu, Mg

[a]RDA, recommended dietary allowances; ESADDI, estimated safe and adequate daily dietary intakes.

Table 14.6. Mean iron intake in France: data from INSEE and from epidemiological surveys

	INSEE (mg/d)	Epid. surveys[a] (mg/d)
Women	10	11.6
Pregnant women	12.5	12.6
Man	13.5	15.8

[a]From Hercberg [12].

Conclusion

The purchasing method is a reliable one for estimation of the mean nutrient content of the average diet of a population.

Nevertheless, this method cannot be a substitute for more precise methods (food intake surveys and relative nutritional status). It warns nutritionists and epidemiologists about risk groups in connection with certain micronutrients, which are more likely to be subdeficient. In this study women seem to be a more exposed group to micronutrient subdeficiencies (fluoride, manganese, iron, zinc, magnesium, copper, calcium, folic acid, vitamins B1, B6 and E).

References

1. Haeusler L (1985/86) La consommation alimentaire: perception et réalité. Centre de recherche pour l'étude et l'observation des conditions de vie. Consommation, 2:3–14
2. Dupin H, Mareschi JP (1984) Habitudes alimentaires – mode de vie et apport nutritionnels: implications technologiques. Colloque du 14 juin 1984 de la Fondation Française de Nutrition, 71 av.Victor Hugo, 75116 Paris. Réalisations 1984, pp 33–44
3. Anonyme (1986) Les Français consomment toujours plus de graisses. Chiffres OCDE. Confluences Diététiques. 43. 68 rue Mazarine, 75006 Paris
4. Beyer MN, Mercier MA (1986) Consommation et lieux d'achat des produits alimentaires en 1982. Collection INSEE, ser. Ménages no. 117, p.100, INSEE, Paris
5. Dupin H (1981) Apports nutritionnels conseillés pour la population française. CNRS-CNERNA. Technique et Documentation Lavoisier
6. Souci SW, Fachmann W, Kraut H (1980) Food composition and nutrition tables 1986/87. Wissenschaftliche Verlagsgesellschaft mbH, Stuttgart
7. Paul AA, Southgate DAT (1978) McCance and Widdowson's The composition of foods. Elsevier-North Holland Biomedical, Amsterdam
8. Darret G, Couzy F, Antoine JM, Magliola C, Mareschi JP (1986) Estimation of minerals and trace elements provided by beverages for the adult in France. Ann Nutr Metab 30:335–344
9. Couzy F, Aubree E, Magliola C, Mareschi JP (1988) Average mineral and trace elements content in daily adjusted menus (DAM) of French adults. J Trace Elem Electrolytes Health Dis 2:79–83

10. Antoine JM, Magliola C, Couzy F, Darret G, Mareschi JP (1986) Estimation of the share of each water source for adults in France. Ann Nutr Metab 30:407–414
11. Anderson GH, Peterson RD, Beaton GH (1982) Estimating nutrient deficiencies in a population from dietary record: the use of probability analyses. Nutr Res 2:409–415
12. Hercberg S (1988) in La carence en fer en nutrition humaine. Editions Médicales Internationales, Paris
13. Mareschi JP, Magliola C, Couzy F, Aubree E (1987) The well balanced diet and the "at risk" micronutrients: A Forecasting Nutritional Index. Int J Vit Nutr Res 57:79–85
14. Mareschi JP, Magliola C, Aubree E, Couzy F (1987) Can the mineral elements intakes recommended for the French population be provided by a balanced diet? Int J Vit Nutr Res 57:225–230
15. Committee on Dietary Allowances, Food and Nutrition Board, National Research Council (1980) Recommended dietary allowances, 9th rev. edn, National Academy of Sciences, Washington, p 123
16. Pennington JAT, Young BE, Wilson DB, Johnson RD and Vanderveen JE (1986) Mineral Content of Foods and total diets: the selected minerals in foods survey 1982 to 1984 J Am Diet Ass 86, 876–91.

CHAPTER 15

Food Additive Intake: Estimated Versus Actual

B.H. Lauer[1] and D.C. Kirkpatrick[1]

The Bureau of Chemical Safety in Ottawa is particularly concerned with safety standards as they apply to chemicals in food, and for purposes of this chapter, the term "safety standard" as it relates to a food additive will be the "acceptable daily intake" (ADI). The ADI is defined as "the dietary intake of an additive which can be safely ingested daily by a human over a lifetime without appreciable risk on the basis of all known facts at the time of evaluation" [1]. The ADI is a figure usually derived from long-term toxicological testing of the additive in laboratory animal species and is normally ascertained by taking a fraction (most often 1/100) of the "No-Observed Adverse Effect Level" (NOAEL) in the most sensitive mammalian species tested. One might argue about the arbitrariness inherent in the ADI concept and in some cases, one might even argue over toxicological interpretations that lead to its estimation in specific cases. Nonetheless, most food regulatory agencies are familiar with this figure and use it as a standard against which "probable daily intakes" (PDIs) or theoretical daily intakes (TDIs) may be compared. The concept of ADIs will not be considered further as the focus of this chapter is on the forecasting and actual measurement of intakes of the additive after an ADI is established and the additive is permitted under national legislation to be used in various foods.

The sweetener aspartame is used as an example to illustrate approaches to intake estimation and determination. In 1981, provision was made in the Canadian Food and Drug Regulations for the use of aspartame as a sweetener and flavour enhancer in a number of foods (Table 15.1). These included table-top sweeteners, breakfast cereals, beverages (including beverage concentrates and mixes), desserts/topping/fillings (including mixes thereof) and chewing gum and breath-freshener products. At the time of initial approval and listing of this sweetener, it was proposed that the use patterns and intake of aspartame be monitored by means of a post-market surveillance program, in order to provide data concerning the distribution of aspartame intake, including the mean and upper

---

[1]Bureau of Chemical Safety, Food Directorate, Health Protection Branch, Health and Welfare Canada Ottawa, Ontario, Canada K1A 0L2.

Table 15.1. Food uses of aspartame approved in Canada

Foods	Maximum permitted level of use
Table-top sweeteners	Good manufacturing practice
Breakfast cereals	0.5%
Beverages, beverage concentrates, beverage mixes	0.1% in beverages as consumed
Desserts, dessert mixes, toppings, topping mixes, fillings, filling mixes	0.3% in product as consumed
Chewing gum; breath freshener products	1.0%

From: Item A.3, Table VIII, Division 16, Canadian Food and Drug Regulations (Part B), Departmental Consolidation of the Food and Drugs Act and of the Food and Drugs Regulations, Canadian Government Publishing Center. Supply and Services Canada, Ottawa, Canada K1A 0S9

percentiles for high users. In practice consumption monitoring for this additive did not actually get under way in Canada until 1987, since sufficient time had to be allowed for products containing it to achieve market penetration.

Methods of Intake Estimation

While awaiting market penetration and the opportunity to undertake actual consumption determinations, several exercises in intake estimation, that is, calculating a theoretical daily intake or TDI, were undertaken. In the case of aspartame, three methods were used, all of which have inherent flaws as they are estimates and no more. But as long as the manner in which they are flawed is recognized then they can serve a useful purpose in the interim period between the time of first approval of an additive and the time of actual consumption monitoring.

Method 1 is only applicable to additives such as sweeteners that are intended to replace basic food ingredients such as sugar. At the time of approval of aspar-

Table 15.2. Aspartame consumption: estimation using Method 1

Annual per capita disappearance of sugar in Canada (1985)[a]	43.07 kg

$$\frac{43070 \text{ g}}{365 \text{ days}} = 118 \text{ g/day}$$

$$1 \text{ g sugar} = 5 \text{ mg aspartame}$$
$$118 \text{ g sugar} = (118 \times 5) \text{ mg aspartame}$$
$$= 590 \text{ mg aspartame}$$
$$\text{Mean adult weight}^{b} = 53.64 \text{ kg}$$
$$\text{Aspartame intake} = \frac{590 \text{ mg/day}}{53.64 \text{ kg}} = 11 \text{ mg/kg b.w./day}$$

[a]From Robbins [2].
[b]Computed from data in Demirjian [3].

Table 15.3. Aspartame consumption: estimation using Method 2

Product	Per capita disappearance[a] (g/day)	Aspartame concentration (ppm)	Aspartame intake (mg/day)
Breakfast foods	8.76	1250	10.95
Soft drinks	191.75	480	92.04
Cocoa	3.36[b]	5160	17.34
Tea	2.68[b]	21750	73.08
Chocolate drink	10.19	300	3.06
Yoghurt	4.95[c]	600	2.97
Ice cream	17.36[c]	800	13.89
Total			213.33

Total aspartame intake = 213.33 mg/day

Mean adult weight = 53.64 kg

$$\text{Aspartame intake} = \frac{213.33 \text{ mg/day}}{53.64 \text{ kg}} = 3.98 \text{ mg/kg b.w./day}$$

[a]From Robbins [2].
[b]Expressed on a dry basis.
[c]Volume statistics converted to mass statistics.

tame, there was no other artificial sweetener approved for use as a food additive in Canada, which made application of this approach somewhat more valid.

The aspartame intake was calculated (Table 15.2) by assuming that aspartame could replace all added sucrose (i.e. as opposed to that which is naturally present). The annual per capita disappearance of sugar in Canada in 1985 was 43.07 kg (118 g/person/day). If approximately 5 mg of aspartame replaces 1 g of sugar, then the aspartame intake would be 590 mg/person/day or approximately 11 mg/kg body weight (b.w.)/day.

What are the flaws in this approach? First, it was assumed that there would be complete replacement of sucrose, even though technologically and realistically, this was unlikely. Thus, the figure tends to be an overestimate. On the other hand, aspartame could be used to replace sweeteners other than sucrose (e.g. glucose solids and high-fructose corn syrup solids). Insofar as these other sweeteners are used in foods that contribute significantly to the total dietary aspartame intake (e.g. soft drinks) the overestimate of intake obtained previously is moderated or counterbalanced by substitution of aspartame for sweeteners other than sucrose, as well as substitution for sucrose itself.

Method 2 made use of per capita disappearance data of major foodstuffs eligible to contain aspartame. The data were obtained from the *Handbook of Food Expenditures, Prices and Consumption* [2]. These data, along with the average aspartame concentration for the designated food products and the resultant aspartame intakes, are shown in Table 15.3. In connection with the food products specified in this table and the aspartame intake estimates, the following should be noted:

1. The per capita disappearance of cocoa was used in the absence of statistics on hot chocolate mix.

2. The intake figure for tea is based on all tea products.

3. Per capita disappearance data were unavailable from this source on drink mixes, freeze pops, puddings, gelatins, toppings, chewing gum and table-top sweeteners.

Taking these considerations into account, this approach yields an estimated aspartame mean intake of 213 mg/person/day, equivalent to about 4 mg/kg b.w./day.

What are the flaws of this approach? First, the results do not take into account atypical consumers or particular segments of the population which may warrant special attention such as infants and children, pregnant women, etc. In addition, individual likes, dislikes, special diets and changing eating habits due to age are disregarded. It should also be mentioned that deriving intake estimates on the assumption that a product is consumed by the entire population results in an underestimate of actual intake.

Method 3 is the most sophisticated of all and in this instance, data on food consumption were derived from the 24-hour dietary recall portion of the Nutrition Canada National Survey [4]. This survey was conducted in Canada in the early 1970s and was designed to determine the prevalence of nutritional diseases in the Canadian population and to identify and determine the quantity of food items consumed by the Canadian public. Some 13000 individuals comprising all ages had medical, dental and anthropometric examinations, in addition to a dietary interview. The sample design permitted consequent evaluations or assessments to be made on the basis of a number of variables including population groups, geographical locations, seasons, age, sex, income levels and pregnancy. The food consumption data were weighted in accordance with the design of the survey to provide population estimates of food consumed for the various age groups. Where food consumption data were not available from the Nutrition Canada Survey, data from other Canadian sources, as well as a number of United States sources, were utilized. For a more specific breakdown of products within the general food categories in which aspartame is permitted, use was made of information provided as part of the aspartame formal food additive petition offered to the Health Protection Branch, as well as information obtained from various food manufacturers and market surveillance data. In many cases, the actual use levels of aspartame in these various food products were obtained directly from food labels, since the Canadian Food and Drug Regulations require that the concentration of this additive on an "as sold" and "as consumed" basis be declared on the labels of food containing it. The foods considered and their actual aspartame levels on an "as consumed" basis are shown in Table 15.4. The specified actual level of use is an average of use levels for different brands of product typically available in the marketplace within each designated product category. With the exception of soft drinks, there was no attempt to weight the average according to production volumes or relative market share of individual brand products. In the

Table 15.4. Level of aspartame in various products[a]

Products that may contain aspartame	Aspartame concentration[b] (ppm)
Breakfast cereals	1250
Beverages[c]	
Soft drinks	480
Hot chocolate mix	401
Iced tea mix	250
Chocolate-flavoured dairy drink	300
Drink mixes	260
Freeze pops	800
Desserts[d]	
Yoghurt	600
Ice-cream analogs	800
Puddings	538
Gelatins	503
Toppings	2100 µg/serving
Confectionery[e]	
Sugar-free gum	4800 µg/stick
Mints	10000[f]

[a] Actual levels of use in products available in the Canadian marketplace.
[b] On "as consumed" basis.
[c] Includes beverage concentrates and beverage mixes.
[d] Includes dessert mixes, toppings, topping mixes, fillings and filling mixes.
[e] Includes chewing gum and breath freshener products.
[f] No actual use levels available; level shown is maximum permitted under Canadian Regulations.

case of soft drinks, it was estimated on the basis of relative consumption of colas versus lemon–lime drinks that cola-type beverages accounted for twice the volume of any other soft drink type. All other soft drink types were assigned a value of 1. In the case of mints, no actual use levels were available, and therefore the maximum permitted level of use under the Canadian Regulations was utilized.

The All Persons Mean Intakes (APMI) (i.e. including eaters and noneaters) and the Eaters Only Mean Intakes of the food products that may contain aspartame for 1–4 year olds (M+F), 12–19 year olds (M) and overall ages groups (M+F) are given in Table 15.5. These age groups were chosen so that the broadest range of aspartame intakes could be captured on both a per capita and body weight basis, without estimating intakes for all age groups and sexes in the population.

Consumption data were obtained from the Nutrition Canada Survey and a number of other sources (Table 15.5) and it should be noted that the intake data are from comparable but not identical age groups. For example, the intake data

Table 15.5. Intake of foods (g/day) by various age groups[a]

	All persons mean intake			Eaters only mean intake		
Product	1–4 years (M&F)	12–19 years (M)	All ages (M&F)	1–4 years (M&F)	12–19 years (M)	All ages (M&F)
Breakfast cereals	3.7	5.4	2.5	21.7	52.1	33.2
Beverages						
Soft drinks	40.0	200.5	106.1	195.6	441.7	360.2
Hot chocolate mix	7.2[b]	14.2 [b]	– [c]	432 [d]	276 [d]	305 [d]
Iced tea mix	9.3	79.3	221.6	134.7	384.9	548.4
Chocolate flavored dairy drink	10.7[b]	61.1 [b]	– [c]	230 [d]	333 [d]	346 [d]
Drink mixes	31.0[e]	41.05[e]	245 [e]	258 [d]	415 [d]	342 [d]
Freeze pops	– [c]	– [c]	– [c]	– [c]	– [c]	– [c]
Desserts:						
Yoghurt	0.9	1.5	1.3	115.2	112.5	144.2
Ice-cream analogs	16.5	29.4	17.6	63.5	116.4	88.7
Puddings	11.7	10.9	9.5	149.6	174.6	149.4
Gelatins	5.0[b]	6.0[b]	– [c]	132 [d]	224 [d]	170 [d]
Toppings	– [c]	– [c]	– [c]	– [c]	– [c]	– [c]
Confectionery						
Sugar-free gum	– [c]	– [c]	– [c]	– [c]	– [c]	– [c]
Mints	4.0[f]	7.0 [f]	4.3[f]	19.3[f]	28.2[f]	26.6[f]
Overall total	140.5	456.3	386.9			

[a]Data obtained from the 24-hour dietary portion of the Nutrition Canada National Survey [4] unless otherwise indicated; all intakes are on "as consumed" basis.
[b]Data obtained from Pennington [5].
[c]No data available.
[d]Data obtained from Pao et al. [6].
[e]Data obtained from USDA [7].
[f]Data based on consumption figures for candy other than chocolate.

from Pennington [5] are for 2-year olds and 14–16-year olds instead of 1–4-year olds and 12–19-year olds. The data from Pao et al. [6] are for 1–2-year olds and 15–18-year olds. The USDA [7] data are for 1–2-year olds and 12–14-year olds. Consumption figures for breakfast cereals are based on intakes of wheat and bran cereals, which were considered representative of breakfast cereal consumption *per se*. In the absence of intake data on mints, consumption figures for candy other than chocolate were used. The iced tea intakes are based on consumption data for all tea.

Prior to examining aspartame intakes, it is instructive to examine Table 15.5 more closely. For all age groups examined, soft drinks are a major contributor to the Total Mean Food Intake of products that may contain aspartame. For 1–4-year olds, drink mixes are also major contributors, such that in combination with soft drinks, these two product categories represent more than 50% of the total mean

Table 15.6. Aspartame consumption: estimation using Method 3

| | All persons mean intake (mg/day (mg/kg b.w./day)) | | |
| | 1–4 years | 12–19 years | All ages |
Product	(M&F)	(M)	(M&F)
Breakfast cereals	4.6 (0.33)	6.8 (0.13)	3.1 (0.06)
Beverages			
Soft drinks	19.2 (1.37)	96.2 (1.88)	50.9 (0.93)
Hot chocolate mix	3.1 (0.22)	5.7 (0.11)	— [a]
Iced tea mix	2.3 (0.16)	19.8 (0.39)	55.4 (1.01)
Chocolate flavored dairy drink	3.2 (0.23)	18.3 (0.36)	— [a]
Drink mixes	8.1 (0.58)	10.7 (0.21)	6.2 (0.11)
Freeze pops	— [a]	— [a]	— [a]
Desserts			
Yoghurt	0.5 (0.04)	0.9 (0.02)	0.8 (0.01)
Ice-cream analogs	13.2 (0.94)	23.5 (0.46)	14.1 (0.26)
Puddings	6.3 (0.45)	5.9 (0.12)	5.1 (0.09)
Gelatins	2.5 (0.18)	3.0 (0.06)	— [a]
Toppings	— [a]	— [a]	— [a]
Confectionery			
Sugar-free gum	— [a]	— [a]	— [a]
Mints	40.0 (2.86)	70.0 (1.36)	43.0 (0.78)
Total intake	103.0 (7.36)	260.8 (5.10)	178.6 (3.25)

[a]No data available.

food intake for this age group. The very substantial contribution (i.e. greater than 50%) of iced tea mix to the all ages Mean Total Food Intake is probably inflated since the estimated intake of this product is based on total tea consumption.

An examination of the mean food intakes of the specified products for the various age groups by all persons (i.e. eaters and non-eaters combined) and eaters only clearly demonstrates the dilution effect of non-eaters on the all persons mean intakes of these products. On the basis of these data, the eaters only mean intakes of products were one to two orders of magnitude greater than the all persons mean intakes. This is an important consideration in assessing exposure to substances, such as high-intensity sweeteners, which are used in foods consumed by particular segments of the population (e.g. dieters, diabetics, etc.).

Table 15.6 shows the all persons mean intakes of aspartame in mg/capita/day and in mg/kg b.w./day for the various age groups. These intakes were derived by multiplying the levels of aspartame in each product (Table 15.4) by the all persons mean intake of that product (Table 15.5).

On the basis of these estimates, soft drinks and mints are major contributors to the total aspartame intake of all age groups examined (i.e. they represent approximately 20%–40% of the total). In the case of 1–4-year olds, ice-cream analogs (which includes fudgesicle-type products) are also a major contributor (13%), followed closely by drink mixes and puddings. For 12–19-year old males, ice-cream analogs contributed approximately 10%, followed closely by iced tea mix and chocolate-flavored dairy drinks. Iced tea mix was also a major contributor to the total APMI for the all ages group (31%), but as noted earlier, this is probably an overestimate. Similarly, the contribution of mints to the total aspartame intake for all age groups is considered to be an overestimate since the maximum-permitted aspartame use level was utilized in this calculation and the food intake data were based on consumption figures for all candy (other than chocolate).

The total All Persons Mean aspartame intakes ranged from 103–261 mg/capita/day (3.2–7.4 mg/kg b.w./day). The highest aspartame mean intake on a mg/capita basis was for 12–19-year old males, but on a body weight basis, was for 1–4-year olds.

As noted previously, a number of assumptions were made in deriving these estimates of aspartame intake. Several of these assumptions can lead to over-estimates. However, there are also a number of factors which moderate the overestimates and, in fact, suggest that these intakes are underestimates. These factors include the following:

1. The effect of including non-eaters in mean intake calculations. On the basis of the data presented herein, this can result in intake estimates that are an order of magnitude too low.
2. The unavailability of food intake data on products that can contribute to the total aspartame intake. As a result, foods such as table-top sweeteners, freeze pops, toppings, and chewing gum were not included in the intake estimates.
3. The impact of changes in consumption patterns. The Nutrition Canada Survey was conducted more than 15 years ago and consumption of certain products such as yoghurt has increased over the years (i.e. on the basis of per capita dis-appearance figures).

Consumption Monitoring Program

Very early in the approval process, in fact, even before aspartame was approved for use in Canada, the Health Protection Branch began to consider the post-market surveillance of this food additive. It was considered that since this type of additive had potential for widespread use, which cut across all food types and user groups, it was important to verify theoretical predictions by undertaking a monitoring program of actual consumption. Such work had never been under-taken in Canada previously and thus, it was desirable to employ proper method-ology and protocols in order to ensure success.

In establishing this type of survey, it was considered that the following topics had to be addressed: method of data-reporting, duration of the study, extent of food monitoring, types of foods to be monitored, the type and size of samples to be employed, whether or not a separate survey for particular target populations (e.g. diabetics) should be conducted, the regions of the country to be included and demographic details, the number of survey "waves" per year, scheduling of the survey waves (i.e. the time of year or season), sample selection, age groups to be included in the survey, methodology to be employed in statistical analysis, procedures taken to reduce errors, and the cost. Obviously, setting out the parameters for such a study proved to be a major activity.

The Canadian Food Industry tabled several proposals. One of these involved the conduct of a market penetration study to determine aspartame consumption by the public-at-large in order to justify a second study which would follow later. The second study, which would target only beverages, was based on the premise that the bulk of aspartame was being used in beverage products and that by examining beverage consumption, one could largely account for aspartame consumption by the population. Concern was expressed over this proposal insofar as it would only measure the intake of beverages, and restricting the study to such products would compromise its usefulness and purpose, particularly in connection with future requests for extensions of use of this additive to foods other than those already listed in the Canadian Regulations. Two other proposals were based on use of an existing consumer mail panel and involved maintaining a food consumption diary. One of the proposed studies was a 7-day national study, and the other was a 14-day study to be undertaken in Ontario and Quebec only. These proposals gave some indication of what was potentially achievable by the industry. By incorporating elements of both, consolidated recommended minimum specifications for a consumption monitoring study were developed.

The main features that the Health Protection Branch wished to see incorporated into a consumption monitoring study may be summarized as follows:

- It would be based on a food consumption diary
- The diary would be kept for at least 7 days
- Those categories of foods containing aspartame would be monitored
- A fixed panel would be employed, supplemented where necessary
- Selected major cities across Canada would be involved
- Two waves (representing summer and winter consumption) would be undertaken
- Each wave would be spread over several weeks and respondents would be randomized to weeks
- Information would be provided by the survey research company on how existing panel members were recruited
- The age groups to be included would be 0–5, 5–9, 10–15, 15–19, 20–35 years (M+F) (i.e. children, teenagers and women of child-bearing age would be included)
- Statistics should include: average daily consumption (mg/kg b.w./day), upper ninetieth percentile of average daily consumption, each decile of average daily consumption, percentage of those exceeding the ADI (all of the foregoing to be calculated for users and the total sample separately for each age/sex category), the frequency distribution of intake, percentage of those consuming the addi-

tive, profiles of the highest users, and an indication of any change between surveys in the level of consumption
- Diabetics should be surveyed as a separate component
- Details should be provided on non-sampling errors, procedures used to reduce
such errors, and estimates of errors from similar surveys

Based on these key features, the NutraSweet Company, the original petitioner
for aspartame, offered a proposal to the Health Protection Branch. It was based
on a 7-day food consumption diary, comprised a summer and winter wave, would
monitor all food categories encompassing aspartame-containing foods, and met
Branch specifications with regard to statistics to be reported. The proposal advo-
cated use of an existing mail panel of 5000 households and the panel would be
balanced to reflect distribution of Canadian families within each region with
respect to such parameters as age of the homemaker, family income and community size. Moreover, the age groups of interest to the Branch would be covered
and in general, the minimum number of individuals, males and females in total,
in each age group met the Branch's specification of at least 500. The study would
also look at special populations such as dieters (i.e. those on weight-reduction
regimes) and diabetics.

Throughout the last part of 1986 and the beginning of 1987, extensive consulta-
tions were held with the NutraSweet Company to finalize this proposal. The major
discussions centered around panel selection procedures, a "singles" supplement to
the panel, and procedures related to non-response and partially completed diaries.

The study was undertaken in 1987 and the Branch had an opportunity to review
the results of the first wave ("cold weather wave"), undertaken in the winter/
spring of that year, and to suggest improvements in data reporting for the consolidated results of the two waves. The results of the two waves have now been
presented to the Health Protection Branch and further interpretation is given by
Heybach and Ross [8].

Wave 1, undertaken from February to April, 1987 comprised 5200 households
(7700 individuals). Wave 2, undertaken from July to September, 1987 comprised
5125 households (7500 individuals). The percentage household return rate for
Wave 1 ("cold weather wave") was 73% and for Wave 2 ("warm weather wave")
was 66%. Diaries were kept by an adult selected within a family household. If
there were children in such households, a child was also selected at random.
Households were predesignated for male or female adult selection initially, in
order to sample disproportionately males because of their lower completion rate.
The study instrument consisted of a questionnaire or diary kept for seven days in
which all relevant consumption of foods and beverages was recorded. The 15
product areas examined were: carbonated soft drinks, powdered drinks, frozen
juices/drinks, hot chocolate/cocoa, milk-based drinks or shakes, iced tea mixes,
hot flavoured teas, puddings/jellos/topping mixes, yoghurt, pie, popsicles,
cereals, gum, hard candies/breath mints, artificial sweeteners, children's vitamins and wine coolers. Respondents were given some flexibility in reporting
data; for instance, drink consumption could be reported in milliliters or any other

identified volumetric unit. Aids were available to assist in reporting data: respondents were provided with a measuring cup, a conversion table (ounces/cups into milliliters), a chart translating the volume of single-serving beverage containers into milliliters, and a list of all brands in relevant food categories along with code numbers to avoid brand identification errors during reporting.

With regard to the "cold weather wave" (CWW), within the various age categories, the APMI (M+F) resulting from "true" food additive use (i.e. food additive use excluding table-top sweeteners) ranged from 0.20 mg/kg b.w./day (64+ years) to 0.81 mg/kg b.w./day (2–5 years). The "overall" (i.e. all ages) APMI was 0.50 mg/kg b.w./day; the eaters only mean intake, 1.15 mg/kg b.w./day; the 90th Percentile APMI, 3.41 mg/kg b.w./day; and the 90th percentile eaters only intake, 5.00 mg/kg b.w./day. Total aspartame consumption figures (i.e. including table-top sweetener use) were slightly higher (0.56, 1.28, 3.79 and 5.54 mg/kg b.w./day, respectively).

With regard to the "warm weather wave" (WWW), the APMI resulting from true food additive use ranged from 0.36 mg/kg b.w./day (64+ years) to 0.85 mg/kg b.w./day (2–5 years). The "overall" APMI was 0.55 mg/kg b.w./day; the eaters only mean intake, 1.21 mg/kg b.w./day; the 90th Percentile APMI, 3.73 mg/kg b.w./day and the 90th percentile eaters only intake, 5.40 mg/kg b.w./day. Total aspartame consumption figures (including table-top sweetener use) are again slightly higher (0.60, 1.32, 4.05, and 5.87 mg/kg b.w./day, respectively).

The APMI figures (all foods and beverages; table-top sweeteners included) for those on a weight loss diet (1.26 mg/kg b.w./day CWW; 1.46 mg/kg b.w./day WWW) and diabetics (1.27 mg/kg b.w./day CWW; 1.90 mg/kg b.w./day WWW) were about twice the overall (all ages) APMI (0.56 mg/kg b.w./day CWW and 0.60 mg/kg b.w./day WWW). The eaters only mean intakes for those on a weight loss diet (1.80 mg/kg b.w./day CWW; 2.04 mg/kg b.w./day WWW) and diabetics (1.88 mg/kg b.w./day CWW; 2.88 mg/kg b.w./day WWW) were about 1.5 times the overall eaters only mean intakes (1.28 mg/kg b.w./day CWW; 1.32 mg/kg b.w./day WWW). The 90th percentile eaters only intakes for those on a weight loss diet and diabetics were comparable, or even lower than similar figures for the general population. The eaters only mean intakes for diabetics (1.88 mg/kg b.w./day CWW and 2.88 mg/kg/day WWW) are only slightly higher than that (1.15 mg/kg b.w.) published by Virtanen et al. [9].

Some interesting and unexplainable geographical observations were revealed in the "cold weather wave" (similar statistics were not available in the "warm weather wave"). The APMI for Quebec francophones was low (0.28 mg/kg b.w./day) compared with Quebec anglophones (0.49 mg/kg b.w./day), the latter being close to the overall population mean intake (0.50 mg/kg b.w./day). On the other hand, Ontario and Alberta consumers were relatively high (0.63 and 0.61 mg/kg b.w./day). Rural consumers were low (0.39 mg/kg b.w./day), urban consumers were high (0.65 mg/kg b.w./day) and singles and/or multiples were unremarkable (0.54 and 0.50 mg/kg b.w./day, respectively).

One of the more unusual statistics to be employed in this study was the base statistic of "eater-days." In this instance, consumption is examined only on those days during which these eaters actually consumed foods containing the sweetener. This statistic should have greater potential to focus on the high consumer than eater statistics, because an eater, in the context of this study, was defined as a person who consumed any aspartame at all during the study. Since each eater's consumption is averaged over the seven days of the study, consumption figures using this statistic as a base tend to be reduced due to the moderating effect of days on which the "eater" does not consume aspartame. If the 90th and 95th percentile data using "total eaters" as a base are compared with those using "total eater-days" as a base, it can be seen that the latter data are somewhat higher, indicating that eaters (as would be expected) did not consume aspartame on all days that the diary was kept. On the other hand, in using eater-days as a base statistic, the intakes of people consuming aspartame on one of the seven days is averaged in with those who are consuming aspartame on all seven days. In other words, there is a certain loss of respondent identity when this statistic is applied. The occasional aspartame consumer may therefore be "dragging down" the intakes of the zealous user, and this fact would be lost in the reporting of an average, even though it is an average for an eater day. The other problem is that an eater who has a low consumption of aspartame by virtue of the fact that he or she derives that intake from consuming low consumption items in the diet may be "dragging down" the consumption figure of eaters consuming high intake items. Thus, while the eater day concept does at least represent an attempt to focus on the high aspartame user, it is a difficult statistic to understand and conceptualize.

The high consumption group in the "eater day" data is the 2–5-year old group (95th percentile figures: 15.61 mg/kg b.w./eater day CWW and 13.08 mg/kg b.w./eater day WWW). These are the highest aggregate levels of consumption recorded in this study and these eater day levels differ somewhat from the total eater (i.e. eaters only) figures (95th percentile figures: 12.26 mg/kg b.w/day CWW and 11.48 mg/kg b.w./day WWW). In this regard, it is interesting to note that the cold weather wave consumption is higher than that of the warm weather wave.

Only one person in the study exceeded the ADI (40 mg/kg b.w./day), a 4-year-old male weighing 15 kg, and he did so on two occasions during the seven day recording period. His average intake during the week was 29 mg/kg b.w./day and on the two days that he exceeded the ADI, his intakes were 42 and 43 mg/kg b.w./day. He had been consuming aspartame via carbonated soft drinks and artificial sweeteners only. The other three cases of highest individual consumption were a 43-year-old female weighing 62 kg (average, 24 mg/kg b.w./day; highest single-day consumption, 32 mg/kg b.w./day), a 3-year-old male weighing 23 kg (average, 23 mg/kg b.w./day; highest single-day consumption, 37 mg/kg b.w./day) and a 6-year-old male weighing 17 kg (average, 12 mg/kg b.w./day; highest single-day consumption, 34 mg/kg b.w./day).

Some of the other groups examined for their aspartame consumption included teenage males (13–17-year olds), women of child-bearing age (18–39-year olds), and seniors (65 years and older). The eaters only means (mg/kg b.w./day) were as follows: teenage males, 0.85 (CWW) and 0.91 (WWW); women of child-bearing age, 1.53 (CWW) and 1.50 (WWW); and seniors, 0.81 (CWW) and 0.95 (WWW). The eater-day means (mg/kg b.w./eater-day) were: teenage males, 1.82

(CWW) and 1.59 (WWW); women of child-bearing age, 2.06 (CWW) and 2.14 (WWW); and seniors, 1.24 (CWW) and 1.37 (WWW).

In conclusion and to give some indication of the extensive database that has been derived from this consumption monitoring program, each wave of this study resulted in 111 tables of statistics and, needless to say, there is a great deal of additional information that may be extracted from the study.

Data from this actual monitoring program are compared to the theoretical intake estimates discussed previously. For those statistics that are comparable (i.e. APMI), the results obtained in this study are lower by one order of magnitude than those estimated previously using the other methods discussed. This shows that the theoretical intakes estimated by the predictive methods were conservative. It is not surprising therefore that the actual APMI measured after market penetration for aspartame are lower than these predicted by the other methods. Furthermore, it is interesting to note that the theoretical intake estimates capture the higher consumption aggregate intakes as determined by these actual intakes. On the basis of this exercise, it would appear that both types of procedures are useful, but that consumption monitoring is essential in situations where the use of an additive is widespread and cuts across all foods and demographic groups of consumers. In such cases, consumption monitoring verifies and refines pre-approval intake estimates of an additive and provides the basis for sound regulatory policy in connection with assessment of potential future extensions of use of the additive in question.

References

1. Lauer BH (1987) Control of food additives in Canada and its implications on protection of public health. Env Health Rev 31:104–111
2. Robbins LG (1984) Handbook of food expenditures, prices and consumption. Supplement. Marketing and Economics Branch, Agriculture Canada, Ottawa, Canada, Department of Supply and Services publication no. 83/3
3. Demirjian A (1980) Anthropometry report. Health and Welfare Canada, Ottawa
4. Health Protection Branch (undated) Nutrition Canada food consumption patterns report. Health and Welfare Canada, Ottawa, Canada
5. Pennington JAT (1983) Revision of the total diet study: food list and diets. J Am Diet Assoc 82:166
6. Pao EM, Fleming KH, Guenther PM, Mickle SJ (1982) Foods commonly eaten by individuals: amounts per day and per eating occasion. Human Nutrition Information Service, Home Economics Research Report no. 44, US Department of Agriculture, Hyattsville, MD
7. Consumer Nutrition Division, Human Nutrition Information Service (1983) Food intakes: individuals in 48 states, year 1977–78. Nationwide Food Consumption Survey 1977–78, Report no. I-1, US Department of Agriculture, Hyattsville MD
8. Heybach JP, Ross C (1989) Consumption of aspartame in the Canadian population. J Can Diet Assoc 50:166–170
9. Virtanen SM, Rasanen L, Paganus A, Varo P, Akerblom HK (1988) Intake of sugars and artificial sweeteners by adolescent diabetics. Nutr Rep Int 38:1211

CHAPTER 16

Pesticide Residues in the United States Diet

P. Lombardo[1]

The United States (US) Food and Drug Administration (FDA), the Environmental Protection Agency (EPA), and the US Department of Agriculture (USDA) have joint responsibility in the area of pesticides. EPA registers or approves the use of pesticides and establishes tolerances if the use of a pesticide may lead to residues in food [1,2]. With the exception of meat and poultry, for which USDA is responsible, FDA is charged with enforcing these tolerances on imported food or domestic food shipped in interstate commerce.

FDA has carried out a large-scale monitoring program for pesticide residues in foods since the 1960s [3]. The program has two principal elements: (a) regulatory (commodity) monitoring, to measure residue levels in domestic and imported foods to enforce tolerances or other legal limits; and (b) the Total Diet Study, to determine dietary intakes of pesticides and other selected chemicals.

Regulatory Monitoring

The prime objective of the monitoring element is to prevent foods that contain illegal pesticide residues from reaching the consumer. As a very important by-product, information is developed on the incidence and levels of pesticide residues in the US food supply. This provides FDA with an overview of the pesticide residue situation in foods, and is a measure of the effectiveness of the US regulatory system. The monitoring results are summarized and made available to EPA, other government and international agencies, and the general public through the scientific literature or other means.

Domestic samples are collected as close as possible to the point of production in the food distribution chain, since the emphasis is on enforcement of tolerances established by EPA. Sampling at an early stage of distribution provides the best

[1]Division of Contaminants Chemistry, Food and Drug Administration, 200 C Street South West, HFF-421 Washington, DC 20204, USA

opportunity to effect timely regulatory follow-up, if such is indicated. Import samples are collected at the point of entry into the US. Mexican shipments are given special attention because of the large volume of fresh and processed foods that enter the US from that country. This is especially true during the winter months, when much of the fresh produce consumed in the US comes from Mexico.

About 18000 shipments of food were collected and analyzed in 1988 [4,5]. Imported foods comprise more than half the total, reflecting FDA's increased emphasis on imports. Shipments from about 80 different countries are sampled each year. The foods are analyzed for a wide variety of possible pesticide residues. Of the approximately 250 different pesticides that would be detected were their residues present, about 110 have been found in recent years [4,5]. There are currently about 300 pesticides with US tolerances on foods, as well as a number of other pesticides and related chemicals that can exist as residues. Because of the great number of possible pesticide–commodity combinations, selective monitoring of foods of dietary importance is carried out to achieve effective consumer protection.

The residue analytical methodology employed is critical [6]. Most analyses are carried out using one of five well-tested and validated multiresidue analytical methods. In combination, these methods can determine about half the pesticides with food tolerances, as well as many of their metabolites, alteration products, and associated chemicals. Single residue methods are used when the residues of interest are not amenable to determination by the multiresidue methods. FDA realized early in its monitoring of foods for pesticide residues that the use of a separate method for each pesticide would require so many analytical resources that adequate monitoring coverage could not be achieved. FDA attempts to maintain uniform limits of quantitation for a given pesticide in all its laboratories. In general, the amount of sample taken for analysis and the instrument sensitivity are adjusted such that a limit of quantitation of about 0.01 ppm for most pesticides is obtained (variable according to the response of the detector to the individual chemicals).

Over the past several years, no residues have been found in more than half the food samples examined, and less than 1% contained residues that exceeded the tolerances. This indicates that pesticides are rarely used in a manner that results in excessive residues. Of the samples with violative residues, about 80% were considered illegal or violative because there was no tolerance for those specific pesticide–commodity combinations, though tolerances exist for other, often similar commodities, frequently at levels significantly higher than those found in the violative sample; the remaining 20% contained residues that exceeded tolerances.

Total Diet Study

The second major element of the FDA pesticide program is the Total Diet Study, a program that has been carried out since the 1960s [7]. This approach, in contrast to the regulatory monitoring described above, provides the means to directly estimate dietary intakes of pesticide residues (intakes of industrial chemicals, heavy metals, radionuclides, and essential minerals are also determined). The principal objectives are to calculate dietary intakes, to compare them with acceptable daily intakes (ADIs) established by scientists at joint meetings of the World Health Organization (WHO) and the United Nation's Food and Agriculture Organization (FAO), and to identify trends. The Total Diet Study also serves as a final check of the effectiveness of the US regulatory system for pesticides.

Foods are purchased at the retail level in supermarkets or grocery stores (just as a typical shopper would do) throughout the US. About 5000 foods were identified as comprising the diet of the US population in two comprehensive nationwide dietary surveys carried out in the 1970s [8,9]. Using an aggregation scheme, 234 foods were selected to represent the 5000 foods [10,11]. Most of these individual 234 foods represent a group of foods similar in type and nutrient content; the food that is analyzed is the group member consumed in the greatest amount. For example, apple pie represents dozens of different fruit pies and pastry with fruit, and spaghetti and meatballs in tomato sauce represents a number of pasta dishes. Diets were constructed for eight different age–sex groups: the 6–11-month-old, the 2-year-old, and 14–16, 25–30, and 60–65-year-old males and females [10]. Dietary intakes for each of these groups can be calculated because each of the 234 foods is analyzed separately. Each year, four "market baskets" composed of these 234 foods are collected. For each market basket, food items are collected in each of three cities in a broad geographic region of the US. The three samples of each food are combined, and the foods are prepared table-ready, i.e., as they would typically be cooked or otherwise prepared in the home. The degree of preparation varies from the very simple, such as peeling bananas, to preparing complex foods such as beef stew or lasagna. The foods are then analyzed using methods capable of identifying and measuring over 100 pesticides, as well as other chemicals. Since the Total Diet Study is conducted to determine the levels of residues in foods as normally eaten, and because the levels of pesticide residues in such foods are usually very low, the analytical procedures used have been modified to permit quantitation at levels five to ten times lower than those achieved in FDA's regulatory monitoring, in the range of 0.001–0.002 ppm for many pesticides. Also, the identity of each pesticide residue found is confirmed by an alternative technique. The dietary intakes are then calculated and compared with the ADIs.

The dietary intakes for the pesticides found in the 1988 study are given in Table 16.1 for the infant, the teenage male, and the older female. As can be readily observed, the intakes are generally manyfold lower than the FAO/WHO ADIs. Current ADIs [12] are listed for reference. ADIs have not been established for all pesticides, and some ADIs include several chemicals which may be related because of their formation during manufacture or as a result of environmental degradation. The DDT (1,1,1-trichloro-2,2-bis(p-chlorophenyl)ethane) group is a good example of the latter; this group includes o,p'- and p,p'-DDT, o,p'- and p,p'-DDE, and p,p'-TDE.

Table 16.1. Pesticide intakes (μg/kg body wt/day) found in Total Diet analyses and their ADIs for three age/sex groups in 1988

Pesticide	FAO/WHO ADI[a]	Age/sex group		
		6–11 months	14–16 year M[b]	60–65 year F[b]
Acephate	3	0.0105	0.0080	0.0104
Azinphos-methyl	2.5	0.0013	0.0039	0.0031
BHC, alpha + beta	–[c]	0.0008	0.0014	0.0010
BHC, gamma (lindane)	10	0.0008	0.0014	0.0009
Captan	100	0.0295	0.0141	0.0359
Carbaryl	10	0.0519	0.0086	0.0124
Chlordane, total	0.5[d]	0.0007	0.0007	0.0010
Chlorobenzilate	20	0.0055	0.0015	0.0011
Chlorpropham, total	–	0.1639	0.2140	0.0976
Chlorpyrifos	10	0.0141	0.0071	0.0061
Chlorpyrifos-methyl	10	0.0125	0.0175	0.0080
DCPA	–	0.0011	0.0009	0.0013
DDT, total	20[d]	0.0681	0.0264	0.0115
DEF	–	<0.0001	<0.0001	<0.0001
Diazinon	2	0.0057	0.0059	0.0033
Dicloran, total	30	0.1868	0.0394	0.0889
Dicofol, total	25	0.0217	0.0066	0.0156
Dieldrin	0.1[d]	0.0114	0.0049	0.0039
Dimethoate	10[d]	0.0077	0.0020	0.0063
Diphenylamine	20	0.0141	0.0417	0.0330
Endosulfan, total	8[d](T)[e]	0.0376	0.0159	0.0224
Endrin	0.2	<0.0001	<0.0001	0.0001
Ethion	6(T)	0.0119	0.0039	0.0033
Fenitrothion	3	0.0014	0.0023	0.0017
Fenvalerate	20	0.0010	0.0006	0.0010
Folpet	10(T)	0.0009	0.0003	0.0011
Fonofos	–	0.0001	0.0001	<0.0001
Heptachlor, total	0.5[d]	0.0040	0.0017	0.0007
Hexachlorobenzene	–	0.0016	0.0011	0.0006
Iprodione, total	300	0.0017	0.0013	0.0014
Linuron	–	0.0025	0.0009	0.0012
Malathion	20	0.1360	0.1332	0.0819
Methamidophos	0.6	0.0126	0.0133	0.0253
Methidathion	5	0.0010	0.0009	0.0007
Methiocarb	1[d]	0.0001	<0.0001	<0.0001
Methomyl	10(T)	0.0026	0.0011	0.0028
Methoxychlor, p,p'	100	0.0003	0.0001	0.0001
Mevinphos, total	1.5[d]	0.0017	0.0008	0.0020
Monocrotophos	0.6	[f]	<0.0001	0.0001

Table 16.1. (*Continued*)

Pesticide	FAO/WHO ADI[a]	Age/sex group		
		6–11 months	14–16 year M[b]	60–65 year F[b]
Omethoate	0.3	0.0024	0.0026	0.0062
Parathion, total	5	0.0073	0.0008	0.0015
Parathion-methyl	20	0.0002	0.0001	0.0002
Pentachlorophenol	–	0.0004	0.0002	0.0003
Permethrin, total	50[d]	0.0376	0.0737	0.1075
Perthane	–	0.0003	0.0001	0.0002
Phorate, total	0.2[d]	0.0001	0.0002	0.0002
Phosalone	6	0.1227	0.0007	0.0007
Phosmet	20[d]	0.0111	0.0032	0.0064
Pirimiphos-methyl	10	0.0002	0.0001	0.0001
Quintozene, total	7[d]	0.0009	0.0016	0.0008
Sulfur	–	0.0090	0.0119	0.0126
Tecnazene, total	10	0.0003	0.0002	0.0002
Toxaphene	–	0.0087	0.0078	0.0116
Triallate	–	0.0001	<0.0001	0.0001
Vinclozolin	40[d](T)	0.0071	0.0033	0.0081

[a]ADIs are usually expressed as mg/kg body wt/day but are expressed here as μg/kg body wt/day for ease of comparison. The ADIs cited here reflect revisions made in 1987.
[b]M = male, F = female.
[c]ADI not established.
[d]Includes other (related) chemicals.
[e]T = "temporary" ADI.
[f]No consumption of a food item containing this residue in this age/sex group.

Of the more than 200 chemicals that can be determined by the procedures used, about 50 are typically found each year. Table 16.2 lists the 30 most frequently found pesticides in 1988 and their frequency of occurrence. Over the past 10 years, malathion and DDT have been the most frequently found pesticides. Malathion is widely used on many grains, fruits, and vegetables, and is found in almost one-fourth of the 234 Total Diet foods. DDT, although no longer permitted for use on foods in the US, continues to be found at very low levels (chiefly as DDE) in many foods, primarily those of animal origin. As can be seen, none of the daily intakes approached established ADIs. Dieldrin is closest with an intake approximately 6% of the ADI for the teenage and adult groups.

Intakes of persistent chlorinated pesticides have declined steadily since cessation of their agricultural uses in the US over a decade ago; however, residues of these pesticides continue to occur at low levels, particularly in foods of animal origin [13]. Although not pervasive, low-level residues of some of the more recently developed pesticides are now appearing. Because these pesticides are generally not as stable as the older chlorinated pesticides, their residue levels in ready to eat foods are low, as are their resulting dietary intakes.

Table 16.2. Frequency of occurrence of pesticides in Total Diet Study in 1988

Pesticide[a]	Total no. of findings[b]	Occurrence (%)
Malathion	242	21
DDT	237	20
Diazinon	171	15
Chlorpyrifos	124	11
Dieldrin	122	10
Chlorpyrifos-methyl	115	10
Endosulfan	89	8
Hexachlorobenzene	86	7
Dicloran	76	6
Methamidophos	63	5
Heptachlor	58	5
BHC, alpha and beta	52	4
Lindane	48	4
Chlordane	46	4
Chlorpropham	40	3
Dimethoate	39	3
Quintozene	39	3
Carbaryl[c]	35	3
Acephate	33	3
Ethion	29	2
Dicofol	27	2
DCPA	22	2
Parathion	20	2
Omethoate	19	2
Phosalone	19	2
Toxaphene	19	2
Permethrin	16	1
Captan	13	1
Chlorobenzilate	12	1
Sulfur	12	1

[a]Isomers, metabolites, and related compounds have not been listed separately; only the generic or "parent" pesticides from which they arise have been included.
[b]Based on 1170 items.
[c]Reflects overall incidence; however, only 72 selected foods were analyzed for N-methylcarbamates.

For a number of analyses, the bulk of the intake is derived from a relatively small number of foods. As examples, about 80% of the malathion intake derives from grain-based products, and about 85% of the carbaryl intake is from fruits [13].

Data from the 1987–88 USDA Nationwide Food Consumption Survey have been received, and a new food list is being created. Consideration is being given to expanding the number of population groups, with a particular focus on children. In addition, the Total Diet Study will be revised to reflect the changes in food consumption.

Summary and Conclusions

No residues were found in more than half the food shipments sampled and analyzed in the regulatory monitoring conducted by FDA in 1987 and 1988. When residues were found, they were usually at low levels and rarely exceeded tolerances. Most violative residues were found in commodities for which a tolerance had not been set for the specific pesticide in question. These findings illustrate that pesticides are rarely used in a manner that results in residue levels that exceed tolerances.

In the Total Diet Study conducted over the past several years, about 50 pesticides are typically found each year. The most frequently found residues are DDE, an environmentally persistent metabolite of DDT, and malathion, an insecticide widely used on fruits, vegetables, and stored products such as grains. The levels of most pesticide residues found were orders of magnitude lower than residue tolerances applicable to raw agricultural commodities established by EPA. This may be attributed in part to the effects of food preparation, such as cooking and washing, on residue levels. Dietary intakes were far below established ADIs.

The Total Diet Study will be revised to incorporate more recent food consumption information, and will continue to serve as a final check on the effectiveness of the US pesticide regulatory system.

References

1. Code of Federal Regulations (1988) Title 21, sections 193 and 561. US Government Printing Office, Washington, DC
2. Code of Federal Regulations (1988) Title 40, section 180.101. US Government Printing Office, Washington, DC
3. Reed DV, Lombardo P, Wessel JR, Burke JA, McMahon B (1987) The FDA pesticides monitoring program. J Assoc Off Anal Chem 70:591–595
4. Anonymous (1988) Food and Drug Administration pesticide program – residues in foods – 1987. J Assoc Off Anal Chem 71:156A–174A.
5. Anonymous (1989) Food and Drug Administration pesticide program – residues in foods – 1988. J Assoc Off Anal Chem 72:133A–152A.
6. Anonymous (1968 and revisions) Pesticide analytical manual, Vols I and II, Food and Drug Administration, Washington, DC
7. Pennington JAT, Gunderson EL (1987) History of the Food and Drug Administration's Total Diet Study – 1961 to 1987. J Assoc Off Anal Chem 70:772–782
8. Nationwide Food Consumption Survey Data Tapes. Spring, Summer, Fall, and Winter Quarters 1977–78, US Department of Agriculture, 1980, 1981. PB-80-190218, PB80-197429, PB80-200223, PB81-118853, National Technical Information Service, Springfield, VA

9. Second National Health and Nutrition Examination Survey, 1976–80. Data Tape 5704 (24-Hour Recall, Specific Food Item), National Center for Health Statistics, 1982. PB82-142639, National Technical Information Center, Springfield, VA

10. Pennington JAT (1983) Revision of the Total Diet Study food list and diets. J Am Diet Assoc 82:166–173

11. Pennington JAT (1981) Documentation for the revised Total Diet Study: food list and diets. PB82-192154, National Technical Information Service, Springfield, VA

12. Anonymous (1987) Pesticide residues in foods – 1987. Report of the joint meeting of the FAO panel of experts on pesticide residues in food and the environment and a WHO expert group on pesticide residues. Food and Agriculture Organization of the United Nations, Rome, Italy

13. Gunderson EL (1988) FDA Total Diet Study, April 1982–April 1984, dietary intakes of pesticides, selected elements, and other chemicals. J Assoc Off Anal Chem 71:1200–1209

CHAPTER 17

Monitoring Dietary Radiocesium Intake in Sweden After the Chernobyl Accident

E.-M. Ohlander,[1] W. Becker[1] and Å. Bruce[1]

Introduction

The accident at the nuclear power station at Chernobyl in the USSR on 26 April 1986 affected not only the Soviet Union, but also many other countries in Europe. Radionuclides were deposited over large areas, where they fell to the ground mainly with rain. Radioactive fallout in Sweden was very unevenly distributed (Fig. 17.1).

In May 1986, the National Food Administration (NFA), in consultation with the National Institute of Radiation Protection, set action levels for the cesium-137 activity in foods sold on the market [1].

In collaboration with other authorities, the NFA organized the analysis of thousands of food samples for radionuclides. The analyses of samples collected during summer 1986 showed increased levels of cesium activity, especially in game, reindeer, freshwater fish, wild berries and wild mushrooms from areas with heavy fallout. Most of these foods do not reach the market and therefore the NFA gave special dietary advice on consumption of such self-sufficiency foods from areas with heavy radioactive fallout [1].

The main objective of the measures taken by the NFA was to ensure that the intake of radioactive substances from foods was kept below a level corresponding to an effective dose equivalent of 5 mSv/capita during the first year and 1 mSv/capita annually during the subsequent years. With the fallout from Chernobyl 1 mSv corresponds to about 50 000 Bq ^{137}Cs/annum (140 Bq/day).

In order to obtain data on the general intake of cesium-137 in different areas of Sweden, and to estimate whether the above goals were reached, several projects were carried through from summer 1986 to winter 1988. In a food basket study a number of foodstuffs bought on seven occasions in eight towns all over Sweden were analyzed to provide basic data for calculation of the collective effective dose equivalents from foods bought on the market [1,2]. In other projects, duplicate portions of servings from schools, canteens and individuals (hunters and fishermen) were analyzed for the cesium-137 content [2].

[1]National Food Administration, P.O. Box 622, S-751 26 Uppsala, Sweden.

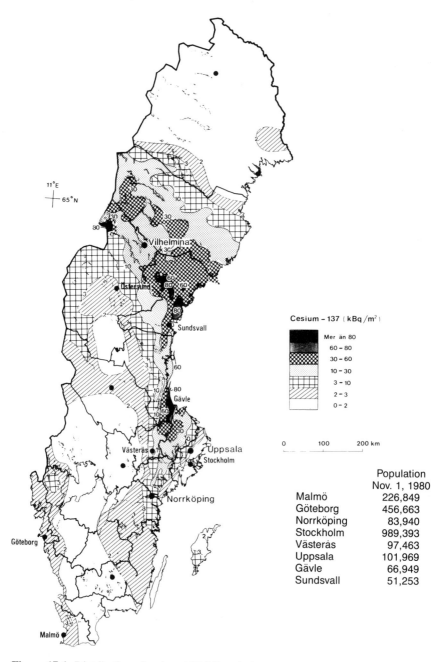

Figure 17.1. Distribution of cesium-137 fallout in Sweden after the Chernobyl accident. Towns (incl. population data) included in the food basket surveys are shown.

Materials and Methods

The Food Basket Study

Selection of Regions

To cover a large part of the population, eight major towns were chosen including both areas exposed to a heavy fallout (Gävle, Uppsala, Sundsvall) and areas that received less (Västerås, Stockholm, Norrköping, Göteborg, Malmö, Fig. 17.1).

Composition and Purchase of the Baskets

The choice of foods included in the basket was based on the consumption statistics from the Swedish Agricultural Market Board using the definite figures for the year of 1983. Although the consumption varies slightly between years, it was thought most correct to choose the latest definite figures as a base. These data give the consumption of foodstuffs combined into groups. In order to produce a shopping list to be used in all the cities alike, the food groups had to be distintegrated into single items. This was done using the Market Board's lists of items constituting each food group and their market shares in relation to each other.

The shopping list consisted of 60 foods and beverages, covering 76% (by weight) of the total annual consumption in kg/capita (Tables 17.1 and 17.2). None

Table 17.1. Solid foods included in the "food basket," average consumption kg/capita/year

Potatoes[a]	65.2	Falu-sausage[a]	5.3	Breakfast cereals	1.8
Sugar	19.9	Meatballs[a]	5.2	Cod, frozen[a]	1.8
Apples[a]	17.0	Beef knuckle[a]	5.0	Liver paste[a]	1.7
Wheat flour	14.6	Cabbage[a]	4.9	Mettwust, smoked[a]	1.7
French loaf	13.9	Chocolate[a]	4.9	Peas, frozen	1.4
Bread, wheat+rye	12.3	Onions[a]	3.9	Peaches	1.4
Eggs[a]	11.2	Chicken[a]	3.9	Cauliflower[a]	1.2
Porkloin[a]	10.7	Butter[a]	3.6	Marshmallows	1.1
Bananas	8.6	Lettuce[a]	3.5	Ham, smoked[a]	0.9
Oranges[a]	8.1	Hot dogs[a]	3.2	Cottage cheese[a]	0.9
Hard cheese[a]	7.7	Lingonberry jam	3.0	Baltic herring[a]	0.9
Ice-cream[a]	6.6	Sweet wheat bread	2.8	Bacon[a]	0.8
Carrots[a]	6.0	Moose meat	2.8	Lamb	0.7
Margarine	5.8	Pasta	2.7	Spinach[a]	0.7
Pears	5.7	Rice	2.7	Beetroot	0.7
Crispbread, rye	5.7	Strawberries[a]	2.7	Cod fillet, fresh	0.6
Tomatoes[a]	5.5	Grapes	2.4		
Cucumber[a]	5.3	Oats, rolled	2.4		
				Total	313.0

[a]Items included in the first basket in June 1986. This basket also included leek, liver and follow-up formula.

Table 17.2. Beverages included the "food basket," average consumption kg/capita/year

Milk, 3% fat[a]	100.4
Lowfat milk, 0.5% fat[a]	46.6
Soft drink[a]	30.8
Beer II, 2.8% alcohol[a]	20.2
Cultured milk, 3% fat[a]	15.2
Small beer, 1.8% alcohol[a]	12.3
Orange juice, ready-to-drink	4.3
Orange syrup, ready-to-drink	3.4
Total	233.2

[a]Items included in the first basket in June 1986.

of the foods are on the average consumed in amounts less than 0.5 kg/capita annually. This basket was purchased in the eight towns in three separate groceries representing the three major wholesale chains. These chains have different deliverers of products and together totally dominate the retail market. At the first collection occasion the shopping list was limited to 33 (Uppsala, Gävle, Sundsvall) or 38 (the rest of the towns) food items believed to have been affected by the fallout. This list was used only once, however. Seven baskets were collected from each shop starting in June 1986 and finishing in December 1987.

In Uppsala the purchase was done by the staff of the NFA and in the other places by those of the local health authorities. The shopper was instructed to select food as an ordinary customer taking advantage of bargain prices, sales etc. within the definitions of the shopping list. The shopper was also asked to choose local products when available. Food items bought were ticked off the list and notes were taken on foods missing. The day of purchase was decided on in advance and the food baskets were immediately transported to the NFA in Uppsala. The shopping list was enclosed.

Duplicate Portion Studies

School Meals

Portions of school lunches from one school in nine towns were collected during one week (five days) in October 1986 and during an additional week in April 1987. The towns were the same as those in the food basket survey and the municipality of Vilhelmina, representing the inland area of Northern Sweden. The amounts of food taken for analysis represented an average of the planned portions for students attending the higher grades of the elementary school and the junior high school. Solid food and beverages were collected separately and immediately frozen at the school. The samples for the whole week were then sent to the NFA by mail.

Restaurant Lunches

Lunch meals from one private restaurant and from one canteen in an office, larger factory or alike were collected during five weekdays in May 1987 in each of the eight towns of the food basket survey. The meal consisted of the main course of the day, including bread, butter, salad and a beverage (usually milk). Solid and liquid foods were collected separately and frozen. The frozen samples were then sent to the NFA by mail.

Individual Duplicate Portions

The diets of ten men living in areas with heavy radioactive fallout and consuming large amounts of freshwater fish, game and wild berries were analyzed for cesium activity. Duplicate portions of the diets were collected during one week in September–October 1986, one in February–March 1987 and one in February 1988. Eight men participated all three times and two men in the first two periods only. One person completed five periods with two additional weeks in December 1986 and in April 1987. Duplicate diets of three Lapps consuming a lot of reindeer meat and freshwater fish were collected during one week in March–April 1987.

Duplicate portions of all foods consumed during the week (including water and beverages) were collected. The participants also recorded what they ate. The portions of game, freshwater fish, wild berries and mushrooms were weighed while the amounts of the other foods were estimated in household measures. Solid and liquid foods were frozen separately and sent to the NFA by mail.

Preparation of the Food Samples

Food Baskets

From each food basket a sample was prepared representing 1% of the annual consumption. When weighing the foodstuffs to be included in the sample, due consideration was given to the fact that the consumption data are based on sales figures including non-edible parts like peels and bones. Therefore, the amount of foodstuff was reduced according to the average percentage of waste for each food item.

The weighed beverages were transferred into a bucket and mixed manually. The solid foodstuffs were minced in a meatmincer and then thoroughly mixed in a food processor. Samples of the fluids and the solids were placed in each of two plastic containers (750 ml). Great care was taken to fill the container to exact volume to ensure correct geometrics when measuring for cesium activity.

Samples of the full-fat milk were also analyzed separately.

Duplicate Portions

The duplicate portions from the school meals, lunch meals and from the individual diets were treated in the same way as the food basket samples. The solid foods were mixed in a food processor and the liquids mixed before samples were transferred into plastic containers, 350 ml and 500 ml, respectively.

Radioisotope Measurements

The gamma emission rates were measured at the Department of Radioecology at the Swedish University of Agricultural Sciences, Uppsala, for 30 minutes with two hyperpure Ge-detectors in a low-background radiation laboratory. (For the first two baskets the time of detection was 10 minutes.) The detectors and the samples were surrounded by shielding consisting of 1 mm copper, 5 cm iron and 10 cm low-active lead. The whole arrangement ensured very low background radiation for counting low activities at high efficiency. The output signals of the detectors were fed into two 4096-channel spectrometry analyzers placed in a separate control room to avoid interference from the operator.

Results

Food Baskets

Food baskets were collected and analyzed on seven occasions from June 1986 to December 1987. The total number of analyses amounted to 336 (i.e. two analyses (fluids+solids) × three shops × eight cities × seven occasions).

Missing Items

The completeness of the collected food baskets was very good. A compilation of food items missing from the individual baskets shows that the percentage of missing items was 2%–6%. The corresponding missing sample weight was less than 1.5%. The food most frequently missing was fresh peaches which were included in the shopping list to represent the group of fresh stone fruits appearing on the market in a very short season. It was missing on 77% of the times it should have been included (i.e. on 168 shopping lists). The next food on this list was moose meat. A large part of this meat is not sold to the consumers through the shops but passed on from hunters directly. Moose was unavailable in 55% of cases. Mutton was missed in 43% of cases due to pronounced market seasons. Fresh cod was missing in 24% of the baskets, most frequently in the four northernmost towns probably because people there have other sources for their fresh fish. Beetroot— fresh, not pickled—was chosen to represent roots other than carrots, but was not available in 10% of cases. It was obvious that fresh herring was almost always available, even though this produce was the next on the "missing list" by 9%. The remaining food items missing such as fresh cauliflower, bananas and oranges, were only occasionally unobtainable.

Calculation of Mean Values

For each basket the six individual figures of cesium-137 activity were compiled into one value representing the basket and city concerned. This was done in the following way. Average figures were calculated, one for the three solid samples

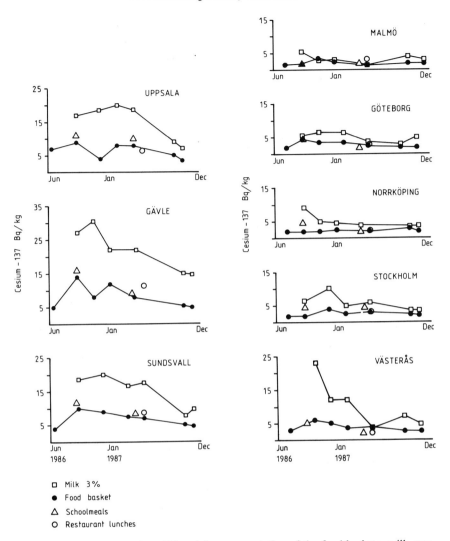

Figure 17.2. Average cesium-137 activity concentration of the food baskets, milk samples, school meals and restaurant lunches during 1986–87.

and one for the three fluid ones using values for the three shops. These two means were weighted together (55% fluids and 45% solids) according to consumption. Table 17.3 shows the results. Both cesium-134 and cesium-137 are listed for solids and fluids plus the average for cesium-137 as described above. These results are also presented in Fig. 17.2 which clearly shows that the cesium activity levels were higher in areas of heavy fallout. The levels increased during the summer of 1986, and then decreased slowly during the autumn and throughout 1987. The occasional drop of the values in the November–December

Table 17.3. Cesium activity concentrations in food baskets (Bq/kg)

City		June 1986 Cesium		September 1986 Cesium			November–December 1986 Cesium			January–February 1987 Cesium			April–May 1987 Cesium			September–October 1987 Cesium			November–December 1987 Cesium		
		137	a	134	137	a	134	137	a	134	137	a	134	137	a	134	137	a	134	137	a
Malmö	Solid	<2	<2	<2	4	2	<2	3.3	3.5	<2	2.7	2.7	<2	2.3	2.2	<2	2.3	2.2	<2	2.3	2.2
	Fluid	<2		<2	<2		<2	3.7		<2	2.7		<2	2.0		<2	2.0		<2	<2	
Göteborg	Solid	<2	<2	<2	4	4	<2	3.3	3.7	1.7	2.7	3.3	<2	2	2.1	<2	2.3	2.2	<2	<2	<2
	Fluid	<2		<2	4		<2	4.3		1.7	4		2	2.3		<2	2.0		<2	<2	
Norrköping	Solid	<2	<2	<2	<2	<2	<2	<2	<2	<2	2.7	2.7	<2	2.3	2.2	2.7	4.0	3.2	<2	2.3	2.2
	Fluid	<2		<2	<2		<2	<2		<2	2.7		<2	<2		<2	2.3		<2	<2	
Stockholm	Solid	<2	<2	<2	<2	2	<2	3	3.9	<2	<2	2.5	<2	2	2.9	1.7	3.0	2.6	<2	2.3	2.2
	Fluid	<2		2	2		<2	5		<2	3		2.3	4		<2	2.0		<2	<2	
Västerås	Solid	<2	3	<2	2	6	1.1	2.6	5.2	<2	2	3.4	2	2	3.8	<2	2.7	2.7	<2	3.0	2.7
	Fluid	4		<6	11		2.4	8.5		2.7	5		3	6		<2	2.7		<2	2.3	
Uppsala	Solid	<2	7	<2	<2	9	1.1	3.1	3.8	2.3	3.3	8.0	<2	2.3	8.0	2	3.3	4.8	2.0	2.7	3.4
	Fluid	12		8	17		3.1	4.7		5.3	13.7		6.3	15.0		2.0	6.7		2.0	4.3	
Gävle	Solid	2	5	2	6	14	<2	3.3	8.0	2.0	6.7	12.1	<2	2.0	8.0	<2	3.7	5.5	2.0	2.0	4.8
	Fluid	9		6	23		7.7	13.7		8.0	18.7		6.3	15.3		3.0	7.7		2.3	8.3	
Sundsvall	Solid	3	4	<2	3	10	1.9	4.9	9.2	2.7	5.7	7.6	2.0	3.3	7.1	2.3	5.3	4.9	<2	2.3	4.6
	Fluid	5		6	19		6.4	14.5		5.3	10		5.3	11.7		<2	4.3		2.7	7.3	

[a]Weighted average of Cs-137 (55% solid + 45% fluid).

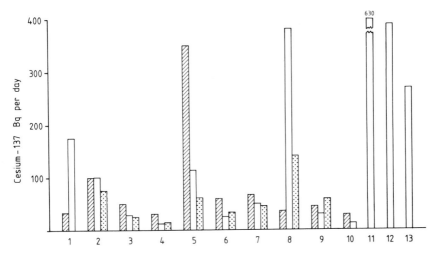

Figure 17.3. Average daily intake of cesium-137 by persons living in areas with heavy fallout and eating large amounts of game, freshwater fish, reindeer during one week in October 1986, February–March 1987 and February 1988. Subjects 1–10 are hunters, subjects 11–13 Lapps.

baskets in Uppsala and Gävle could be due to the fact that a shorter detection time was used.

School Meals

The cesium activity was generally low (Table 17.4). In areas with low levels of radioactive fallout the cesium-137 activity was below 10 Bq/kg and below 5 Bq/portion. In towns with heavy radioactive fallout (Uppsala, Gävle, Sundsvall and Vilhelmina), the levels were higher in milk, 20–40 Bq/l, than in other components. The radioactivity per portion was 6–13 Bq cesium-137/portion, somewhat lower in 1987 than in 1986.

Restaurant Lunches

The cesium activity of the restaurant lunches were also low and on a level similar to that in school meals (Table 17.4). The levels were higher in areas with heavy radioactive fallout, mostly due to the higher activity in the milk.

Individual Duplicate Portions

The cesium activity of the duplicate portions varied considerably between the individuals and the different periods (Fig. 17.3). The mean intake during the week varied from 10 Bq Cs-137/day to 630 Bq/day. For six of the subjects the intake was lower during the second (1987) and third (1988) period than during

Table 17.4. Activity of cesium-137 in school meals during one week in September–October 1986 and April 1987 and in restaurant lunches during one week in April 1987

Town	Period	Cs-137 Bq/kg in		Bq/serving[c]
		Main dish[a]	Beverages[b]	
Malmö				
School	1986	2	2	<2
	1987	2	<2	<2
Restaurant[d]	1987	2	2	2
Göteborg				
School	1986	4	7	3
	1987	<2	4	2
Restaurant	1987	2	4	2
Norrköping				
School	1986	7	4	4
	1987	<2	3	<2
Restaurant	1987	2	4	<2
Stockholm				
School	1986	4	7	3
	1987	<2	9	3
Restaurant	1987	4	4	3
Västerås				
School	1986	5	3	2
	1987	2	<2	<2
Restaurant	1987	<2	2	<2
Uppsala				
School	1986	3	23	7
	1987	3	20	6
Restaurant	1987	4	14	6
Gävle				
School	1986	7	36	9
	1987	2	26	6
Restaurant	1987	4	26	10
Sundsvall				
School	1986	6	23	9
	1987	5	16	8
Restaurant	1987	6	18	8
Vilhelmina				
School	1986	17	19	13
	1987	9	20	9

[a]Including butter, bread, salad etc.
[b]Mainly milk.
[c]Including beverages.
[d]Average of meals collected at a private restaurant and a canteen at a work-site.

Table 17.5. Calculated energy and nutrient content of the food baskets and total per capita supply of foods

Nutrient	Food basket	Per capita supply 1983
Energy (MJ)	11.4	12.0
(kcal)	2727	2871
Protein (g)	91	85
Fat (g)	96	126
Carbohydrates (g)	367	350
Retinol equiv (mg)	1.35	1.8
Thiamin (mg)	2.0	1.8
Calcium (g)	1.2	1.2
Iron (mg)	18	19

the first (1986) period. For two subjects the intake was at a similar level in 1986 and 1987, whereas the intake was substantially higher during 1987 than in 1986 for other two subjects. For these the intake was lower in 1988.

Discussion

The composition of the food baskets was based on the Swedish food balance sheet data. All major foods consumed in Sweden were represented. To check the representativity of the food baskets, the energy and nutrient content were calculated using composition data from the Swedish food tables. The results showed that the content of both energy and nutrients in the baskets were similar to the calculations based on the total per capita supply of foods (Table 17.5). The level of fat was somewhat lower in the food baskets which was mainly due to the fact that margarine was slightly underrepresented. However, the analytical data had shown that margarine was not a source of radiocesium.

The cesium activity of the food baskets varied according to the level of ground fallout (Fig. 17.1). The regional differences in cesium activity of the baskets were to a large extent due to differences in the cesium activity of milk (Fig. 17.2).

In areas with heavy fallout there was a clear decreasing trend in cesium activity after summer 1986. An adult consuming about 2 kg of food per day would have ingested 10–20 Bq cesium-137/day (3–7 kBq/year) in areas of heavy fallout and less than 6 Bq/day (1–2 kBq/year) in areas with small fallout.

The intakes assessed from the food baskets were about half those calculated from food intake data and analytical data for various foods during the first 6 months after the accident [2]. This is probably due to an overestimation of the general cesium level in most foods on the market.

The calculated average yearly effective dose equivalents during the first two years for an adult consuming 2 kg of the food basket foods are shown in Table 17.6. The calculated doses were about twice as high as doses assessed from mea-

Table 17.6. Effective dose equivalents during the first and second year after the Chernobyl accident calculated from the cesium activities of the food baskets

Town	Effective dose equiv.	
	1st year	2nd year
Low fallout		
Malmö	0.04	0.04
Göteborg	0.05	0.03
Norrköping	0.03	0.04
Stockholm	0.05	0.04
Västerås	0.08	0.05
Heavy fallout		
Uppsala	0.13	0.09
Gävle	0.18	0.10
Sundsvall	0.14	0.09
Weighted average[a]	0.06	0.04

[a]According to population.

surements of the whole-body content of radiocesium in a representative sample of Swedes [3]. This could be due to the fact that the whole-body measurements were done on one occasion whereas the food baskets represented intake over a longer period. Moreover, there are also data indicating that dose estimations based on intake data are higher than estimations from whole-body measurements (Becker, Falk and Olofsson, unpublished data).

The food baskets represent the contribution of radiocesium from foods bought on the market. In areas with heavy fallout the cesium intake from game, reindeer, freshwater fish, berries and mushrooms obtained by other means might be substantial. The analyses of the duplicate portions from persons with a great consumption of such foods showed that their cesium intake was in general considerably higher than was calculated from the food baskets.

Assuming that the duplicate portions represented the habitual diet of the hunters throughout the whole study period the intake of cesium corresponded to an effective dose equivalent varying from 0.2 to 1.9 mSv/capita during the first year after the accident and from 0.1 to 1.0 mSv during the second year. For the three Lapps the calculated doses were 2.4–5.5 mSv during 1987. The calculated effective dose equivalents found in this study are in agreement with results from whole-body measurements of persons living in areas with heavy fallout. [4].

Intake of Radiocesium in Some Other Countries

Table 17.7 shows the calculated dietary intake of cesium-137 during the first year after the accident in some countries compared with the Swedish intake data

Table 17.7. Estimated annual intake of cesium-137 (kBq/capita) in some countries during the first year after the Chernobyl accident

Country	Average intake	Special groups
Sweden	3[a] (1–7)	56[b] (5–230)
	7[c] (2–15)	
Norway [5]	9[d] (5–23)	54[d] (10–365)
Finland [6]	10[c] (9–12)	–
West-Germany [7]	3[c]	–
Austria [8]	24[c]	–

[a]Food basket survey.
[b]Duplicate portion study.
[c]Calculated from food balance sheet data and cesium-137 levels in individual foods.
[d]Calculated from food intake data from dietary surveys and cesium-1317 levels in foods.

[5–8]. These data indicate that the general dietary intake of radiocesium after the Chernobyl accident has been moderate in Sweden.

These data are supported by results from measurements of whole-body content of radiocesium (Table 17.8). The whole-body concentration of cesium-137 in the general population was higher in Norway and Finland than in Sweden [3–9]. However, the whole-body data for reindeer-herding Lapps indicate that the intake of radiocesium in this group was higher in Norway and Sweden than in Finland.

General Conclusions

After the accident in Chernobyl several activities were started in Sweden to assess the dietary intake of radiocesium in the population and thereby the effec-

Table 17.8. Whole-body content of cesium-137 in population groups in Sweden, Norway and Finland 1986–1987

Country	Whole-body content (Bq/kg body weight)		
	Areas with low fallout[a]	Areas with heavy fallout[a]	Reindeer herders
Sweden	6[b]	18[b]	390[c]
Norway	15[d]	37[d]	350[d]
Finland	30[e]		170[e]

[a]Average for men and women.
[b]Falk et al. [3].
[c]Olofsson (unpublished data), measurements Jan–Oct 1987.
[d]Bøe et al. [5]
[e]Rahola and Suomela [9].

tive dose equivalent from food. The results of the food basket survey showed that the intake of radiocesium from foods bought on the market was moderate and that it followed the general geographical distribution of the radioactive fallout. The food basket survey proved to be a convenient method of assessing the average dietary intake of radiocesium from foods bought on the market. To assess individual variations in intake and the intake of groups at risk other methods such as dietary surveys or whole-body measurements are needed.

Acknowledgments. The food basket survey was supported by grants from the National Institute of Radiation Protection. On behalf of the National Food Administration we want to thank the staff at the local health authorities for their help with the purchase of the food baskets. We also thank Christina Normark and Clary Pousette, National Food Administration, for preparation of the samples.

References

1. Bruce Å, Slorach SA (1987) Dietary implications of radioactive fallout in Sweden following the accident at Chernobyl. Am J Clin Nutr 45:1089–1093
2. Becker W, Bruce Å, Ohlander E-M (1986) Cesium i kosten (English summary: Cesium in the diet). Vår Föda 38:543–551
3. Falk R, Eklund G, Östergren I (1988) Cesium-137 aktiviteten i Sveriges befolkning två år efter Tjernobylolyckan (Cesium-137 activity in the Swedish population two years after the Chernobyl accident). Paper presented at the Fifth Nordic Symposium on Radioecology, 22–25 August, Rättvik, Sweden
4. Olofsson L, Svensson H (1988) The Chernobyl accident. Transport of radionuclides to man living in northern Sweden. Acta Oncol 27 (Fasc. 6b):841–849
5. Bøe E, Trygg K, Berteig L *et al.* (1988) Stråledose fra mat til menneske etter Tsjernobyl (English summary: Effective dose equivalent from food to man after Chernobyl). SNT-rapport 2, Statens næringsmiddelstilsyn, Oslo
6. Rantavaara A (1988) Radiocesium in domestic foodstuffs in Finland 1986–1988. In: M Kulmala, S Luokkanen, P Aspila (eds) Symposium on Chernobyl fallout studies, Helsinki 9.12.1988. Finnish Association for Aerosol Research, Report Series in Aerosol Science, Helsinki, no 7, pp 11–16
7. Diehl JF, Ehlermann D, Frindik O, Kalus W, Müller H, Wagner A (1986) Radioaktivität in Lebensmitteln – Tschernobyl und die Folgen. Berichte der Bundesanstalt für Ernährung. Bundesforschungsanstalt für Ernährung, Karlsruhe, Dezember
8. Umweltbundesamt (1986) Tschernobyl und die Folgen für Österreich. Bundesministerium für Gesundheit und Umweltschutz, Wien, November
9. Rahola T, Suomela M (1988) Radiocesium in Finns – changes since the 1960's. In: M Kulmala, S Luokkanen, P Aspila (eds) Symposium on Chernobyl fallout studies, Helsinki 9.12.1988. Finnish Association for Aerosol Research, Report Series in Aerosol Science, Helsinki, no 7, pp 17–20

CHAPTER 18

Estimating the Dietary Intake of Veterinary Drug Residues

G.B. Guest[1] and S.C. Fitzpatrick[1]

Introduction

The Codex Committee on Residues of Veterinary Drugs in Foods (CC/RVDF) is an intergovernmental body which advises the Codex Alimentarius Commission on all matters relating to veterinary drug residues. One of the primary objectives of the CC/RVDF is to elaborate maximum residue levels (MRLs) for veterinary drug residues in edible animal products. An important consideration in this process is the acceptability of Codex MRLs from a consumer safety point of view, i.e., having the assurance that Codex MRLs would not result in dietary exposure to residues that exceed the veterinary drug's acceptable daily intake (ADI).

A definitive answer as to whether an ADI has been exceeded can only come from dietary intake studies. A dietary intake study determines the actual daily intake of residues by consumers on the basis of laboratory analysis of food commodities in trade or in consumer channels.

Although a dietary intake study is recognized as the preferred and most realistic way of determining dietary exposures to veterinary drug residues, these studies are expensive, and time-consuming, and may not be feasible if the drug has not been in use for some time. Additionally, dietary intake studies are limited as to the number of commodities and analytes which can be sampled.

Therefore, before the CC/RVDF considers undertaking dietary intake studies on veterinary drug residues, it should attempt to predict whether there is a realistic possibility that use of Codex MRLs for veterinary drugs will result in a dietary intake of a compound that exceeds its ADI.

In 1987, a joint WHO/FAO Consultation on Predicting Dietary Intake of Pesticide Residues (the Consultation) was held in Geneva. The Consultation adopted guidelines to enable national authorities to estimate the dietary intake of various pesticides in their countries. A stepwise procedure for calculating increasingly refined estimates of the dietary exposure to a pesticide residue was proposed.

[1]Center for Veterinary Medicine, Department of Health and Human Services, US Food and Drug Administration, Rockville, MD 20857, USA.

This approach for estimating residue intake can be modified to predict the dietary exposure of veterinary drug residues.

Definition of Terms

The ADI for a veterinary drug is an estimate of the amount of residue of that compound that can be ingested daily over a lifetime without appreciable health risk. The ADI is based upon a complete review of the available data (biological, metabolic, pharmacological, toxicological, etc.) from a wide range of experimental animal studies and/or available relevant human data. The ADI is expressed on a body weight basis.

The CC/RVDF has defined the MRL as the maximum concentration of residue resulting from the use of a veterinary drug (expressed in mg/kg or µg/kg on a fresh weight basis) that is recommended by the Codex Alimentarius Commission to be legally permitted or recognized as acceptable in or on food.

The MRL is based on the type and amount of residue considered to be without any toxicological hazard for human health as expressed by the ADI, or on the basis of a temporary ADI that utilizes an additional safety factor. It also takes into account other relevant public health risks as well as food technological aspects.

When establishing an MRL, consideration is also given to residues that occur in food of plant origin and/or the environment. Furthermore, the MRL may be reduced to be consistent with good practices in the use of veterinary drugs and to the extent that practical analytical methods are available.

ADIs and MRLs for veterinary drugs are calculated for the CC/RVDF by the Joint FAO/WHO Expert Committee on Food Additives (JECFA). The JECFA is composed of internationally recognized experts in the field of veterinary medicine and serves as a scientific advisory body to the CC/RVDF. It meets on an

Table 18.1. Recommended ADIs and MRLs

	Acceptable daily intake	Maximum residue level
Zeranol	0–0.5 µg/kg	10 µg/kg (bovine liver)
		2 µg/kg (bovine muscle)
Albendazole	0–0.05 mg/kg	0.1 mg/kg (muscle, fat, milk)
		5 mg/kg (liver, kidney)
Sulfamethazine	0–0.004 mg/kg	0.3 mg/kg total residue (muscle, liver, kidney, fat)
		0.1 mg/kg parent drug (muscle, liver, kidney, fat)
		0.05 mg/kg total residue (milk)
		0.025 mg/kg parent drug (milk)
Trenbolone acetate (TBA)	0–0.02 µg/kg	2 µg/kg β TBA (muscle)
		10 µg/kg α TBA (liver)

ad hoc basis to evaluate available toxicology and residue data on veterinary drugs considered by the CC/RVDF to be priorities from a public health standpoint.

The JECFA has met twice to evaluate veterinary drug residues. The first meeting took place in Rome in June 1987. The second meeting was held in Geneva in February 1989. The JECFA has recommended ADIs and MRLs for several veterinary drugs (Table 18.1).

Food Consumption Data and Assessment of Risk

The purpose of predicting the dietary intake of a veterinary drug is to compare this prediction with the ADI which was established by the JECFA for that compound. One key factor in making these predictions is a knowledge of the amount of edible animal products consumed.

The collection of valid food consumption data is the most difficult problem to overcome before any assessment can be made about the dietary intake of a veterinary drug residue. Patterns of food consumption vary considerably within individuals and groups of individuals. This is particularly true for food consumption data at the international level where dietary habits are influenced by such factors as ethnic origin, religion, economics and climate.

At its 1989 meeting, the JECFA considered which food consumption values would be representative of edible animal product consumption on an international basis. In order to protect all segments of the population, the JECFA concluded that it would use exaggerated intake data for individual edible tissues and products of animals. It recommended the use of the following food consumption data: 300 g of muscle meat, 100 g of liver, 50 g of kidney, 50 g of fat, 100 g of egg, and 1.5 liters of milk. These food consumption factors apply to all species of food-producing animals.

In the United States, the FDA has traditionally taken a conservative approach to food consumption and considered the 90th percentile consumer when estimating exposure to residues. The 90th percentile consumer eats two to three times more than the average (50th percentile) consumer.

The 90th percentile and the 50th percentile data for edible animal products are shown in Table 18.2. These data are from the 1977–78 Market Research Corporation of America (MRCA) food consumption survey of 11150 individuals over a 14-day period. MRCA provided the data to FDA under contract. Since the survey reports only frequency of eating a particular food item, it cannot be used independently to determine food quantities consumed. To determine the quantity of food consumed, the average portion size was established from a 1977–78 United States Department of Agriculture survey. These data can be used by the United States to predict the dietary exposure of a particular compound on a national basis.

Prediction of veterinary drug residue intake can be made with different degrees of realism. By starting with the most exaggerated intake predictions first, it is possible to eliminate at an early stage, those veterinary drug residues whose intake will clearly not exceed the ADI. A more realistic prediction using more

Table 18.2. MRCA food consumption data

	90th percentile	50th percentile
Bovine muscle	155 g	100 g
Bovine liver	20 g	10 g
Swine muscle	95 g	45 g
Swine liver	10 g	5 g
Poultry[a] muscle	65 g	35 g
Poultry[a] liver	15 g	10 g

[a]Poultry consists of chicken plus turkey data.

refined estimates would make it possible to eliminate other veterinary drugs from further consideration.

Theoretical Maximum Daily Intake

The Theoretical Maximum Daily Intake (TMDI) is a very crude estimate of dietary intake of a compound. For veterinary drugs, it can be calculated by multiplying the Codex MRL by the food consumption values recommended by the JECFA

$$\text{TMDI (mg/kg body wt)} = \frac{\text{MRL} \times 0.3 \text{ kg}}{60 \text{ kg person}}$$

where 0.3 kg is the JECFA food consumption estimates for muscle meat. This results in a prediction of veterinary drug residue intake on the international level. In order to compare the TMDI with the ADI, the TMDI is divided by 60 kg, the weight of the average person.

The TMDI will be a gross overestimation of the true veterinary drug residue intake because:

1. Veterinary drugs are usually not approved in all species of food-producing animals
2. In those species in which a veterinary drug is approved, the percentage of animals treated with the drug is usually far less than 100%
3. Exaggerated values are used for the food consumption of edible animal products
4. Very few edible animal products contain residues at the highest permitted level.

For these reasons it should not be concluded that a proposed Codex MRL is not acceptable when the TMDI exceeds the ADI. However, if the TMDI does not exceed the ADI, further predictions of veterinary drug residue intake are not necessary.

Estimated Maximum Daily Intake

The Estimated Maximum Daily Intake (EMDI) is a more realistic estimate of veterinary drug residue intake. It takes into account the fact that veterinary drugs are usually not approved in all species of food-producing animals.

$$\text{EMDI (mg/kg body wt)} = \frac{\text{MRL} \times \text{90th percentile data from approved species}}{60 \text{ kg person}}$$

The EMDI is calculated by multiplying the MRL by the 90th percentile national food consumption data from the species in which the veterinary drug is approved. In order to compare the EMDI with the ADI, the EMDI is divided by the weight of the average person.

The EMDI is still an overestimation of the actual veterinary drug residue intake because:

1. In those species in which a veterinary drug is approved, the percentage of animals treated is usually far less than 100%
2. The 90th percentile consumer represents the "heavy eater" of meat and usually consumes 2–3 times more than the 50th percentile consumer
3. Very few edible animal products contain residue at the highest permitted level

Estimated Daily Intake

The Estimated Daily Intake (EDI) is the best estimation of veterinary drug residue intake because it takes into account the following factors:

1. Food consumption data for the average consumer
2. Measured residue levels
3. Percentage of animals treated

The EDI is calculated by multiplying the actual residue level (measured from supervised trials, monitoring data, etc.) by the 50th percentile food consumption data from the species in which the veterinary drug is approved. This number is then multiplied by the percentage of animals actually treated with the drug. In order to compare the EDI with the ADI, the EDI is then divided by 60 kg, the weight of an average person.

$$\text{EDI (mg/kg body wt)} = \frac{\text{known residue level} \times \text{50th percentile data} \times \% \text{ animals treated}}{60 \text{ kg person}}$$

Calculations of Dietary Intake

As an illustration of how these guidelines will enable the CC/RVDF to predict the dietary intake of veterinary drug residues, the TMDI, EMDI and EDI will be calculated for two compounds, zeranol and albendazole.

The JECFA established an ADI of 0–0.5 µg/kg for total residues of zeranol. MRLs for bovine muscle and liver were calculated to be 2 µg/kg and 10 µg/kg, respectively.

Appendix 18.1 illustrates the calculations for TMDI, EMDI and EDI for zeranol residues in bovine muscle meat. Even using the worst case assumptions contained in the TMDI equation, the dietary exposure of consumers to zeranol residues is unlikely to approach the ADI. Appendix 18.2 demonstrates similar calculations made for zeranol residues in bovine liver. Comparison of these rough estimates of dietary exposure to zeranol residues with the recommended ADI for the compound provides reassurance that the Codex MRLs are acceptable from a public health standpoint.

The TMDI, EMDI and EDI for albendazole residues in bovine muscle and liver can also be calculated. The JECFA has recommended an ADI of 0–0.05 mg/kg for albendazole. It has established MRLs for total residues of albendazole in the muscle and liver of treated beef cattle of 0.1 and 5 mg/kg, respectively. The JECFA recommends that a 10-day withdrawal period be adhered to when using albendazole.

Appendixes 18.3 and 18.4 illustrate the TMDI, EMDI and EDI calculations for albendazole in bovine muscle and liver, respectively. The results of these predictions indicate that it is highly unlikely that dietary exposure to residues of albendazole would ever approach the calculated ADI for the compound.

Conclusion

Concern has often been expressed in national and international forums over the possible adverse health effects of veterinary drug residues in food. The MRLs established for residues of veterinary compounds may result in residues in edible animal products which exceed the ADI. By establishing guidelines which would enable countries to predict the dietary intake of veterinary drug residues in the various populations in their country, national authorities will be able to provide reassurance that the levels of veterinary drugs in the diet do not pose a threat to health.

Use of these equations to predict the dietary intake of zeranol and albendazole has demonstrated that the MRLs established by the CC/RVDF are very conservative. Adoption of these MRLs by national authorities will not result in unsafe residues in the food supply.

Appendixes

Appendix 18.1: Zeranol Residues in Bovine Muscle Meat

$$\text{ADI} = 0\text{--}0.5 \ \mu g/kg$$
$$\text{MRL} = 2 \ \mu g/kg \ \text{muscle}$$

$$\text{TMDI} = \frac{2 \ \mu g/kg \times 0.3 \ kg^a}{60 \ kg} = 0.01 \ \mu g/kg$$

2% of the ADI

$$\text{EMDI} = \frac{2 \ \mu g/kg \times 0.155 \ kg^b}{60 \ kg} = 0.0052 \ \mu g/kg$$

1% of the ADI

$$\text{EDI} = \frac{0.13 \ \mu g/kg^c \times 0.1 \ kg^d \times 0.25^e}{60 \ kg} = 0.000054 \ \mu g/kg$$

0.01% of the ADI

[a] JECFA value for muscle consumption.
[b] MRCA 90th percentile consumption data for bovine muscle.
[c] Total residues of zeranol in muscle; data from radiotracer studies submitted in New Animal Drug Application.
[d] MRCA 50th percentile consumption data for bovine muscle.
[e] Approximate percentage of animals entering foodchain which have been implanted with zeranol.

Appendix 18.2: Zeranol Residues in Bovine Liver

$$\text{ADI} = 0\text{--}0.5 \ \mu g/kg$$
$$\text{MRL} = 10 \ \mu g/kg \ \text{liver}$$

$$\text{TMDI} = \frac{10 \ \mu g/kg \times 0.1 \ kg^a}{60 \ kg} = 0.017 \ \mu g/kg$$

3.4% of the ADI

$$\text{EMDI} = \frac{10 \ \mu g/kg \times 0.02 \ kg^b}{60 \ kg} = 0.0033 \ \mu g/kg$$

0.67% of the ADI

$$\text{EDI} = \frac{8.2 \ \mu g/kg^c \times 0.01 \ kg^d \times 0.25^e}{60 \ kg} = 0.00034 \ \mu g/kg$$

0.07% of the ADI

[a] JECFA value for liver consumption.
[b] MRCA 90th percentile consumption data for bovine liver.
[c] Total residues of zeranol in liver: data from radiotracer studies submitted in New Animal Drug Application.
[d] MRCA 50th percentile consumption for bovine liver.
[e] Approximate percentage of animals entering foodchain which have been implanted with zeranol.

Appendix 18.3: Albendazole Residues in Bovine Muscle Meat

$$\text{ADI} = 0\text{--}0.05 \text{ mg/kg}$$
$$\text{MRL} = 0.1 \text{ mg/kg muscle}$$

$$\text{TMDI} = \frac{0.1 \text{ mg/kg} \times 0.3 \text{ kg}^a}{60 \text{ kg}} = 0.0005 \text{ mg/kg}$$

1% of the ADI

$$\text{EMDI} = \frac{0.1 \text{ mg/kg} \times 0.155 \text{ kg}^b}{60 \text{ kg}} = 0.00026 \text{ mg/kg}$$

0.52% of the ADI

$$\text{EDI} = \frac{0.05 \text{ mg/kg}^c \times 0.1 \text{ kg}^d \times 0.3^e}{60 \text{ kg}} = 0.000025 \text{ mg/kg}$$

0.05% of the ADI

[a]JECFA value for muscle consumption.
[b]MRCA 90th percentile consumption data for bovine muscle.
[c]Total residues of albendazole in muscle at 10 days withdrawal; 20 mg/kg dose; data from radiotracer studies submitted in New Animal Drug Application.
[d]MRCA 50th percentile consumption data for bovine muscle.
[e]Approximate percentage of animals entering foodchain which would be treated with albendazole.

Appendix 18.4: Albendazole Residues in Bovine Liver

$$\text{ADI} = 0\text{--}0.05 \text{ mg/kg}$$
$$\text{MRL} = 5 \text{ mg/kg liver}$$

$$\text{TMDI} = \frac{5 \text{ mg/kg} \times 0.1 \text{ kg}^a}{60 \text{ kg}} = 0.008 \text{ mg/kg}$$

16.7% of the ADI

$$\text{EMDI} = \frac{5 \text{ mg/kg} \times 0.02 \text{ kg}^b}{60 \text{ kg}} = 0.0017 \text{ mg/kg}$$

3.4% of the ADI

$$\text{EDI} = \frac{3.57 \text{ mg/kg}^c \times 0.01 \text{ kg}^d \times 0.3^e}{60 \text{ kg}} = 0.00018 \text{ mg/kg}$$

0.36% of the ADI

[a]JECFA value for liver consumption.
[b]MRCA 90th percentile consumption data for bovine liver.
[c]Total residues of albendazole in liver at 10 days withdrawal; 20 mg/kg dose; radiotracer data submitted to the New Animal Drug Application.
[d]MRCA 50th percentile consumption data for bovine liver.
[e]Approximate percentage of animals entering foodchain which would be treated with albendazole.

CHAPTER 19

Do Actual Intakes Ever Equal Potential Intakes?

C.E. Fisher[1] and J.A. Norman[1]

Introduction

A variety of methods is available for estimating the intake of chemicals from the diet. A division may be made between those methods which measure, by chemical analysis, the actual intake either of individuals or the "average" consumer, for example duplicate diet and total diet studies, and those which estimate potential intakes either by constructing hypothetical scenarios, for example per capita estimates or by combining food consumption data with concentration data supplied by food manufacturers. This latter method may give actual intakes if there is no degradation of the chemical during storage or subsequent preparation in the home. Even within the same basic study method there are a number of variables which may influence the final intake figure [1]: the analytical method used and assumptions made about concentrations which are below the limit of determination of the analytical methodology, the degree of preparation of the food, whether concentration data are available for all brands of a processed food etc. Although it is, therefore, only possible to estimate actual intakes, with care it is possible to achieve a reasonable approximation to the real situation.

The estimation of potential intakes involves developing reliable models of consumption of the foods in which the chemical of interest is found. Such estimates show what intakes people might achieve but the question which needs to be answered is "do the figures for potential intake which these models yield bear any relation to the intakes people actually have?" This chapter considers to what extent dietary surveys measure "actual" intake, how far estimated potential intakes reflect the actual situation and the implications these questions have when estimated intakes are used to check whether safety standards are being met. The question of whether there are simpler means of determining whether safety standards are being satisfied is also addressed.

[1]Food Science Division MAFF, Ergon House, c/o Nobel House 17 Smith Square, London SWIP 3JR, UK.

To What Extent are Actual Intakes Measured by Analytical Methods?

In a duplicate diet study, individual participants put aside a duplicate of a whole or part (if only particular foods are of interest) of their diet which can subsequently be analyzed for the chemical of interest. Thus for each participant there should be a record of "actual" intake of that chemical during the study period. However, even in this type of study there are problems, principally in determining whether the measured intakes are representative. There are two aspects to this. First, is the duplicate diet which is collected a true representation of what people really ate or did the act of measuring consumption change it? Second, was the short period covered representative of longer-term habits?

There is much evidence to suggest that people actually eat less than normal when participating in a duplicate diet study. This is true even of food scientists who might be expected to appreciate the importance of keeping accurate records of normal habits. Stockley [2] describes a duplicate diet study carried out over a 16-day period. The food scientists experienced a significant loss of body weight during the study period but regained weight after the duplicate diet study was completed. There is also evidence to suggest that people put aside less food than they actually consume. The Ministry of Agriculture, Fisheries and Food (MAFF) undertook a study of fish consumption in conjunction with mercury intake. The study was in two parts, a 4-week diary study of fish consumption and, in the final week of the diary study, a duplicate diet study of the fish component of the diet. There were no major changes in the reported fish consumption during the first three weeks of the dietary study. However, in the fourth week there was a sharp, statistically significant fall in reported fish consumption and, furthermore, the mean weight of the duplicate diets was significantly less than the mean weight of the diary diets (Table 19.1).

The question of whether the short period of a study is a good guide to longer-term intake is more difficult to answer. With a large study population the full range of dietary habits for all ages, important since dietary habits may change over the course of a lifetime, would be represented and hence the measured intakes would give an adequate representation of longer-term intake, unless there are significant changes in external factors. For example the introduction of new

Table 19.1. Fish consumption estimated by a four-week diary study and a one-week duplicate diet study

	Mean fish consumption (g per week)			
	Week 1	Week 2	Week 3	Week 4
Diary study	560 ± 32[a]	500 ± 29[a]	520 ± 31[a]	430 ± 27[a]
Duplicate diet study	—	—	—	350 ± 26

[a]Standard error of the mean.

foodstuffs onto the market may result in a decrease in consumption of previously consumed dietary items. However, duplicate diet studies are time-consuming and costly to carry out and so, in practice, the numbers of participants will be kept as low as possible while ensuring that the study population is statistically representative of the population group of interest.

Duplicate diet studies are concerned with intakes by individuals. Total diet studies, on the other hand, are concerned with the intake of the "average" person and the question arises as to how far this hypothetical "average" person corresponds to the population average. In the UK intakes of heavy metals, pesticides and nutrients by the "average" consumer are estimated by means of the yearly UK Total Diet Study. Information on food consumption is gathered by means of a survey of food purchases by a nationally representative sample of UK households. Food purchased and eaten outside the home, alcoholic drinks and confectionery are not included in the survey. After making allowance for wastage of food, the information collected is used to build up a picture of the "average" person's diet. Samples of the foods making up this hypothetical diet are purchased at a number of locations in the UK (usually about 25); enough food for one complete diet is bought in each place. The foods are prepared, cooked as if for eating and finally combined into groups for chemical analysis. Each food group contains like foods combined together in the proportions in which they are consumed. After analysis, intake of the chemical from each food group is calculated and summed to give the total dietary intake. This does not seem a promising method of measuring actual intake: the consumption data are based on purchase not consumption; some foods and drinks are excluded and only a small number of diets are analyzed. Nonetheless when the results for intake of lead derived from the Total Diet Study are compared with those from a duplicate diet study there is good agreement. In 1982 MAFF carried out a "control" duplicate diet study which was designed to act as a bench mark for lead intake by a population not exposed to any known source of lead contamination. The study population consisted of women and preschool age children. The women's lead intakes can be compared to that estimated for the "average" person for the UK Total Diet Study. In 1982 lead intake by the average woman (person) was estimated to be 0.30 mg per week. The "control" duplicate diet yielded a mean intake for the women of 0.31 mg of lead per week. The limitation of the Total Diet Study, however, is that it cannot give any information on the range of intakes to be found within the population.

However, in some situations, total diet studies cannot give an accurate guide to intake. This happens principally when concentrations of the chemical of interest are below the limit of determination of the analytical methodology. In this situation a number of assumptions can be made about the actual concentration of chemical in the sample

1. That it is equal to the limit of determination: this leads to an upper bound figure which is an overestimate of actual intake
2. That it is equal to zero: This leads to a lower bound figure which is an underestimate of actual intake

3. That it is equal to any arbitrarily chosen value between zero and the limit of determination (most often half the limit of determination)

The inaccuracy of the estimate is obviously compounded if the contributions from a number of food groups in which the concentrations are below the limit of determination are summed.

The Estimation of Potential Intakes Using Hypothetical Scenarios

There are two situations in which estimates of potential intake might be made: (1) it may be necessary to predict what the intake of a chemical will be, for example, when considering the approval of a new food additive it is necessary to predict which types of foods will contain the additive and whether these foods will be widely consumed; (2) if data on the intake of the chemical of interest are only available for the "average" person, it will be necessary to estimate intake of the chemical by the non-average person in order to determine whether all of the population is protected by nationally or internationally agreed safety standards. It is thus necessary to hypothesize as to what intakes "non-average" individuals might have in order to determine how intake by the population as a whole compares with the safety standards. The two situations differ in that in the first case it is necessary to predict which foods will be eaten in significant amounts by significant numbers of people once the additive is permitted, based only on a knowledge of what type of foods the additive might be used in, whereas in the second case it is already known which foods are marketed containing the chemical and it is the variations in dietary habits between individuals which determine the range of intakes within the population.

In situation (1) regulators are forced to assume that all the foods which might potentially contain the chemical of interest will enter the marketplace. This is unlikely to happen in practice and the situation is additionally complicated by the fact that each product is unlikely to be equally successful with each individual in the population. Thus this means of measuring potential intake will greatly overestimate actual intake. This conclusion is borne out by a survey of sweetener intakes by the UK population with special reference to young children and diabetics (J.A. Norman, unpublished). In this study all participants kept a diary of their consumption of foods containing the sweeteners which are permitted in the UK. As well as using these data to calculate their actual intakes of individual sweeteners, some general conclusions about patterns of usage of sweetener-containing products were drawn. When the survey was carried out, the major vehicles in the diet for sweetener intake were soft drinks (both ready-to-drink and concentrates) and yoghurt, both of which were usually labelled as "diet," and table-top sweeteners. In order to estimate potential intake of sweeteners it would be reasonable to assume that people might consume each type of product each day; if individuals are dieting they may try to reduce calorie intake from all sources where there is an alternative available. In practice such a model overestimates intake for all but a small, atypical section of the population because it is based on two fundamental flaws; individuals do not in general consume all possible types of product and even those products which they do consume are not necessarily eaten every day. To make an estimate of the average intake of the population, some measure of the frequency of consumption of the different foods and drinks must be introduced, either by using individuals' consumption data collected via a diary study or by using national consumption data to represent the dietary habits of the "average" person.

Estimates of Potential Intake Using Information Provided by Food Manufacturers

It is difficult to determine intake of food additives analytically since they may be present in only a few brands of a limited number of different types of food and therefore may only be present in duplicate diet or total diet samples at concentrations below the limit of determination of available analytical methods. Thus intakes of food additives must be determined either by using hypothetical scenarios as described above or by combining data on the concentrations of the additive in types of food or brands of a particular food with food consumption data.

Concentration data could be obtained by analyzing individual foodstuffs in the state in which they are consumed but such an exercise is likely to be expensive and time consuming. It may, therefore, be preferable to obtain the information directly from food manufacturers. In the MAFF sweeteners survey, since there was only a small number of sweeteners to consider in relatively few types of food, concentration data were obtained for each individual brand. However, for food colors collecting such detailed data would involve a prohibitive amount of work. When estimates of colors intake were made by MAFF in 1977 [3], information was available on the level of pure dye in each of the foods (or groups of foods) in which the color was used, the total annual usage of each color in particular foods, and other colors which might be used in those foods. Intakes were estimated by constructing three model diets of colored foods (that of the "average" consumer, of a child and of an extreme consumer) based on national food consumption data. These consumption data were combined with the average level of use of each of the foods or drinks to give a daily intake of each color. However, such an estimate assumes that all the colored foods contain the same color which is unlikely to be the case in reality. It is thus a potential estimate rather than an estimate of actual intake. To obtain a more realistic daily intake figure a correction factor was introduced to reflect the intake of colors by people who consume a complete cross-section of colored foods. This correction factor was, for each color, the total annual usage of that single color in each commodity expressed as a fraction of the total annual usage of all colors in that food or drink. Using Yellow 2G as an example, Table 19.2 shows that the "corrected" intake was substantially less than the uncorrected intake. In effect, the uncorrected intake was an extreme case rather than the "average" case the consumption data would suggest.

Table 19.2. Daily intake of Yellow 2G estimated by (1) assuming all colored foods contain the same color and (2) making allowance for the actual usage of each color

Food	All colored foods contain the same color (uncorrected intake mg/day)	Allowance made for actual usage of each color (corrected intake mg/day)
Canned vegetables	2.55	1.15
Chocolate and sugar confectionery	0.79	<0.005
Dry mixes (other than dessert mixes)	0.12	<0.005
Pickles and sauces	1.87	0.18
Soft drinks	3.67	0.04
Total	8.99	1.38

Compliance with Safety Standards

While the model for estimating potential intakes based on the assumption that a person consumes each type of food and drink each day does not represent the majority of the population it does represent a subgroup which is important when it comes to matters of food safety. Governments have a duty to protect the health of all of their citizens not just those who share the dietary habits of the "average" person. Thus the so-called extreme consumer – a person who eats a larger than average amount of the food(s) containing the chemical of interest – is always considered when comparing the intake of the chemical with safety standards. However, it is not easy to obtain data on extreme intake – how does one identify people who consume above average amounts of a freely available food in order to ask them to participate in a duplicate diet or diary record study?

Work within MAFF has shown that it is possible to estimate extreme consumption of an individual food or group of similar foods from a knowledge of the average consumption [4,5]. There exists a simple relationship between a defined measure of extreme consumption and the arithmetic mean consumption of the food by consumers of that food, for example the 90th percentile equals twice the mean consumption by consumers. However, these relationships cannot be applied to the estimation of intake from combinations of different foods because extreme consumption of one food may restrict the choice of consumption of others. Thus there is a problem in estimating even potential intake of a chemical if it is found in a number of foods.

In view of the difficulties involved in making realistic estimates of average and extreme intakes which can then be compared to safety standards such as the FAO/WHO JECFA Acceptable Daily Intakes (ADI) or Provisional Tolerable Weekly Intake (PTWI), much effort has been expended in trying to establish a simple rule-of-thumb whereby it can be ensured that no-one in a population can exceed the ADI or PTWI for a particular chemical. The Danish Budget Method [6], which has been applied to food additives, has been proposed as such a rule-of-thumb. This method is based on the philosophy that although what a person consumes may vary from day to day, the total amount consumed will be roughly constant. Thus the total amount of food or drink consumed can contain an amount of the chemical equal to the JECFA ADI for that chemical. If no individual food or drink contains levels higher than this, the ADI cannot be exceeded so long as the total national constant food or drink consumption is not exceeded. Where the additive is present in both food and drink, the ADI must be apportioned between the two. In actually applying the method the following additional assumptions are often made:

1. That only half the food consumed will be processed and therefore contain additives

2. That products of meat, milk, fish, poultry, vegetables are kept free of additives and so only half the amount of processed foods contain additives

3. In the case of beverages, additives are assumed to occur only in soft drink.

Applying the Danish Budget Method a maximum permissible level in food and a (different) maximum permissible level in beverages can be determined for each chemical for which there is an ADI. These levels could be used as a basis for legislation or, if legislation already exists, to assess whether the statutory limits allow the potential for individuals to exceed the ADIs for any additive. However, it has already been shown that although the potential to exceed an ADI might exist, actual intakes within the population will be much lower than potential intakes. The main drawback of the Danish Budget Method is that it gives no means of knowing whether any individuals in the population are even approaching the ADI; if none are, then it is pointless to set statutory limits based on levels derived using the Danish Budget Method. A more appropriate use for the Danish Budget Method seems to be as a means of prioritizing chemicals for further consideration of intake; if the use levels determined by the Danish Budget Method are close to or lower than current statutory limits or known levels of use, then data on actual intakes need to be collected in order to see whether the ADI is exceeded by any section of the population and, if it is, what proportion of the population is implicated.

Conclusions

Some dietary survey methods such as diary studies, duplicate diet studies and, in some special cases, total diet studies, which estimate intakes by individuals at a certain point in time can be thought of as providing a guide to "actual" intake of a chemical within a population. Potential intakes, that is a guide to the intake which people within a given population might have, are estimated using hypothetical models and on the whole tend to overestimate actual intake. However, when comparing intakes with safety standards special groups in the population must be taken into account.

References

1. Norman JA (1987) How comparable are published data on lead and cadmium intakes. Environmental Health 20 Trace elements in human health and disease: extended abstracts from the second Nordic symposium, 17–21 August, Odense, Denmark. pp 196–199
2. Stockley L (1985) Changes in habitual food intake during weighed inventory surveys and duplicate diet collections. A short review. Ecol Food Nutr 17:263–269
3. Ministry of Agriculture, Fisheries and Food (1979) Food Additives and Contaminants Committee interim report on the review of the colouring matter in food regulations 1973, FAC/REP/29, HMSO
4. Sherlock JC, Walters CB (1983) Dietary intake of heavy metals and its estimation. Chem Ind July:505–508
5. Coomes TJ, Sherlock JC, Walters CB (1982) Studies in dietary intake and extreme food consumption. R Soc Health J 102:119–123
6. Hansen SC (1979) Conditions of use of food additives based on a budget for an acceptable daily intake. J Food Protection 42:429–434

CHAPTER 20

Packaging Materials

L.L. Katan[1]

Introduction

The evaluation of a food contamination toxic hazard involves in principle two components: estimation of human exposure to a contaminant substance, and assessment of the substance's toxicity. Many difficulties arise in estimating exposure to direct food additives or environmental contaminants, but, at least, quantification at source is not a major problem. For packaging materials, however, contamination is indirect, i.e. it involves the extra stage of transfer from packaging materials to food. This is migration.

Thus, to assess hazard it is necessary to know (a) amount of migrant in a food or group of foods, and (b) dietary data in terms of packaging.

(a): The hypothetical maximum amount that could be ingested is, of course, all of the migrant in the package, which is usually known or can be estimated. However, using this is normally a gross overestimate and would lead to the unwarranted rejection of packaging materials which are, in practice, perfectly satisfactory. A large amount of research has been carried out in this field [1–7] and some correlations developed [8–11] but there is still no generally applicable framework from which unit intakes can be estimated.

(b): Some surveillance studies on specific migrants or groups of migrants have been carried out, e.g. vinyl chloride monomer arising from PVC contact [12], plasticisers arising from PVC [13]. These are reliable, but (i) inevitably only give information at a particular date, and (ii) are costly in money and resources. Indeed, it would be totally impracticable to cover a major selection, let alone all packaging materials, in this way.

Estimates have been made, e.g. proportion of packaging materials used in contact with certain types of food, as in guidelines for US legislation [14] and European Community regulations [15]. These have all been based on food consumption statistics for large and crude food groups, typically aqueous–acidic–alcoholic–fatty/oily; and often incorporate major elements of uncertainty caused

[1]14 Field View Drive, Little Totham, Essex CM9 8ND, UK.

by large safety factors. In general, estimation of dietary data in terms of packaging has been a neglected area of research.

The UK Ministry of Agriculture Fisheries and Food has, therefore, set up two major research programs, recommended and supervised by its Working Party on Chemical Contaminants. The first covering (a) is developing a physical–mathematical model of migration, and the first phase of the study has been reported [16]. The second covering (b) is reported here.

Remit and Scope

The project was carried out between 1987 and early 1989 by Maurice Palmer Associates, Cambridge, UK. The objective was to provide an estimate of consumer exposure to different types of primary retail packaging, analyzing the exposure in terms of individual type of food contact surface. It was accepted that the project would include establishment of methodology prior to development of the data.

Obviously, it was desirable to have data as up-to-date and reliable as possible; and the latter criterion dictated calendar year 1986 in order to align with and use the latest National Food Survey (NFS) [17] and, automatically, cover all seasons.

The scope of the study included all types of material used for retail packaging covered by the NFS. Retail packaging was defined to include all materials and articles used for the packaging of food intended for human consumption and included in the NFS, which are in direct contact with the product and purchased by the consumer. Thus, in addition to packaged foods not covered by the NFS, all forms of downstream, industrial, transit and secondary packaging are excluded. Also, closures and their coatings are not included in the presently reported survey. The NFS covers about 250 categories of food; the present survey 115. However, many of the NFS categories describe foods which differ insignificantly from a packaging point of view, and the results apply to the totality of foods covered by the NFS. Taking all the exclusions into account, it is estimated that approximately 85% of total human exposure to packaged food in the UK is covered.

Methodology

Essentially, there are three components.

1. Packaging statistics
2. National diet statistics
3. Merging of points (1) and (2)

As already mentioned, data for component (2) were available from the NFS, and this will not be described further.

Packaging Statistics

Food packaging statistics is a very difficult group of data to develop. Reasons include:

1. Very little packaging is sold by retail as such; consumers purchase filled packages, and hence point-of-sale statistics usually apply to the food, not the package
2. Wholesale statistics for packaging frequently do not distinguish between food packaging and other end uses
3. Data on raw material consumption or use is of very limited use, because the amount used for individual packages varies greatly with size and design; and many raw materials, from tinplate to plastics, enjoy several other applications
4. Price vs. volume correlations vary widely

Hence a wide range of well-recognized market research techniques has been used. These include desk research, shelf audits and a wide range of telephone and in-depth personal interviews with manufacturers and end users of packaging. Where data were not otherwise available, individual packs were measured for weight and surface area. The contractor's prior knowledge of packaging markets, acquired through substantial involvement with the industry over the past 12 years, together with their database, made a substantial contribution to the successful gathering of the statistics.

Data were thus developed for a large number of packages of specific type (size, material, form) containing specific foods. In the following, cream, which was part of a preliminary phase (covering milk products) to establish methodology, will be used for illustration. A characteristic set of basic data for cream in plastic pots is shown in Table 20.1.

Merging

The results for annual consumption were transferred to a spread sheet as shown in Table 20.2. The total for all types of packaging for a particular food must be 100% of the consumption of that food, and hence the individual consumptions

Table 20.1. Basic data: cream (plastic pots), UK, 1986

Pack size As sold (fluid ounces)	SI (ml)	Material[a]	Number of units (millions)	Surface area (cm²)	Pack weight (g)	Total annual consumption (liters)
5	142	PS	10	152	6	1420
5	142	PP	45	152	6	6390
10	284	PS	6	246	13	1704
10	284	PP	45	246	13	12780

[a]PS, polystyrene; PP, polypropylene.

Table 20.2. Merged data: cream (plastic pots), UK, 1986

Total annual consumption (liters)	%	Individual consumption (ml/capita/pack)	Surface area exposure (cm²/capita/year)	Pack weight exposure (g/capita/year)
1420	6	27.4	29.3	1.1
6390	29	123.4	132.1	5.2
1704	8	32.9	28.5	1.5
12780	57	246.7	213.7	11.3
	100	430.4		

Table 20.3. Combined data: cream (NFS Code 17), UK, 1986

Descrip-tion	Unit size As sold	SI	Material[a]	Coating	Individual consumption (ml/capita/pack)	Surface area exposure (cm²/capita/year)	Pack weight exposure (g/capita/year)	Coating exposure (cm²/capita/year)
Fresh and UHT								
Rigid plastic	5 fl. oz.	142 ml	PS		27.4	29.3	1.1	
Rigid plastic	5 fl. oz.	142 ml	PP		123.4	132.1	5.2	
Rigid plastic	10 fl. oz.	284 ml	PS		32.9	28.5	1.5	
Rigid plastic	10 fl. oz.	284 ml	PP		246.7	213.7	11.3	
Carton	1 pint	568 ml	Paper/PE		109.7	81.5	3.9	
Rigid plastic	Portion	10 ml	PS		22.4	75.6	5.6	
Brick pack	200 ml	200 ml	Paper/Al/PE		57.9	66.0	2.6	
Aerosol	250 ml	250 ml	Metal		86.9	119.5	38.9	
Flexible	1 pint	568 ml	PE		54.8	93.0	0.7	
Frozen								
Sterile can	6 oz.	170 g	Steel	Lacquer	72.2	78.6	14.0	78.6
Sterile can	10 oz.	283 g	Steel	Lacquer	54.6	53.1	8.3	53.1
Total					888.9	970.9	93.1	131.7

[a]PS, polystyrene; PP, polypropylene; PE, polyethylene; Al, aluminum foil.

calculated for each pack type, using NFS data. From this, the surface area and packaging weight exposure could be calculated, as shown. Corresponding figures can then be summed for a given product in a given pack or material, as shown in Table 20.3.

Discussion

In a novel study relating to a large number of consumer choice factors, operating on a large human population, it is not surprising that many preliminary difficulties arose and many errors were possible and approximations needed. Indeed, there is little doubt that substantial intrinsic variability exists from one population group to another, even in the same country. Doubtless, such variations would be larger from country to country and year to year.

The NFS covers solid foods and some important liquid foods, e.g. milk, but excludes beverages and some other liquid foods. As already mentioned, it is estimated that the survey applies to approximately 85% of total diet.

With respect to the pack itself, two difficult problems relate to (a) proliferation of plastics, and (b) composites. Concerning (a) there are not only many more polymer types to identify than were in use for food packaging even ten years ago, but even within a polymer type very significant grade variations exist. Copolymers complicate the matter further. For the present survey, it was decided to group plastics by main monomer only, i.e. (polypropylene) (PP) covers all copolymers of propylene containing > 50% of this monomer. However, low-density polyethylene (LDPE), linear LDPE (LLDPE) and high-density polyethylene (HDPE) are distinguished, as well as very well-established copolymers such as polyacrylonitrile-butadiene-styrene (ABS) and polystyrene-acrylonitrile (SAN).

With respect to (b) composites, it may be necessary, in the future, to delve deeper, but for the moment they have been dealt with as follows:

- Metal cans: identified as coated or uncoated
- Metal foil: identified by nature of metal (usually aluminum)
- Plastic composites (laminates): all plies identified where possible; if not, at least proximate ply (in contact with food) identified
- Paper composites: all plies identified where possible; if not, at least the proximate ply (in contact with food) identified

There are many borderline situations where it is not obvious whether products should be covered or not. Examples include packaging film sold as such and used in the home; food consumed away from the home (not included in the NFS); and food wrapped at the retail outlet. Other, even more subtle, questions arise with items such as egg cartons and apple trays – contact or not? As a rule these were excluded so that the survey could be said accurately to cover retail packaging.

Conclusion

The work is being extended to the food categories (mainly beverages) and retail packaging (mainly closures) not covered above, and it is hoped to update it periodically. Now that the methodology, including appropriate computer programs, has been established, this will be less onerous than the initial studies reported. There will then be available a periodically updated series of statistics giving exposure of the average UK population member to migration from retail food packaging. Combining these with estimates of migration per unit pack will enable migration exposure risk to be quantified with much greater accuracy and, more importantly, reliability than in the past. The first use to which the data will be put is prioritization of research on specific aspects, but in due course it may well fit into the framework for development of regulations. Since these are increasingly based on EC (European Community) Directives [18] it will, presumably, be necessary to develop corresponding data for the EC.

Finally, it is recognized that basing any regulatory action on data applicable to average population members must imply deviation for any given individual. This, however, is a problem general to all aspects of dietary intake data, and refinements (e.g. for special risk groups, such as children) for the present topic will follow corresponding changes in more general aspects, e.g. the NFS itself. The main extension of the study envisaged for the future is extension into the food supply chain prior to retail packaging, e.g. bulk transport, storage and processing, and subsequent to it, e.g. domestic hollowware and cookware, home packaging, kitchen utensils, etc.

Acknowledgements. I am indebted to Mr. M. Palmer, Miss S. Garnham and members of MPA staff for invaluable assistance. The work forms part of a research project sponsored by the UK Ministry of Agriculture Fisheries and Food to whom thanks are also due. The results of the research are the property of MAFF and are Crown copyright.

References

1. Klahn J, Figge K, Freytag W (1981) Migration of low molecular packaging components into food. Dtsch Lebensm-Rundsch 7:241–254
2. Smith LE, Chang SS, Senich GA (1981) Migration of low molecular weight additives in polymers. NBSIR Report 81-2314, Washington, DC
3. Karcher W, Haesen G, LeGoff B (1983) Survey of migration studies. Report no. EUR 8286 EN, CEC, DG for Science, Research and Development, EC Luxembourg
4. Adcock LH (1984) Model migration studies. Plastics Rubber Proc Appl 4:53–62
5. Brun S (1983) Materials in contact with food. CNERNA colloquium, Paris, 9–11 February

6. Di Lorenzo C, Vito-Colonna M (1985) Paper and plastic packaging for food products: the migration phenomenon and analytical methods. Ente Nazionale per la Cellulosa e per la Carta, Rome, publication no. 25. 119 pp

7. Ashby R, vom Bruck CG (eds) (1988) Fifth international symposium on migration. Food Add Contam 5: Suppl

8. Garlanda T, Masoero M (1966) Chim Ind 48:936

9. Reid RC, Schwope AD, Sidman KR (1983) Proceedings of the Fourth International Symposium on Migration, Hamburg

10. Katan LL (1979) Plastics Rubber Mats Applics 1979:4,18

11. Katan LL (1981) Plastics in Retail Packaging Bull 4 (9), 7; 3 (7), 5

12. Anonymous (1978) Survey of vinyl chloride content of PVC for food contact and of foods. Food surveillance paper no. 2. MAFF, London, HMSO

13. Anonymous (1987) Survey of plasticiser levels in food contact materials and in foods. Food surveillance paper no. 21. MAFF, London, HMSO

14. Anonymous (1988) Recommendations for chemistry data for indirect food additives petitions. Food and Drugs Administration, Division of Food Chemistry and Technology, Center for Food Safety and Applied Nutrition, Department of Health and Human Service. Washington, DC 20204

15. Directive 85/572 of 19 December 1985. Official Journal of the European Community, L372/14 of 31 December 1985

16. Chatwin PC, Katan LL (1989) The role of mathematics and physics in migration prediction. Packaging Technol Sci 2 (2), 75

17. Anonymous (1986) Household food consumption and expenditure. Annual report of the national food survey committee. MAFF, London, HMSO

18. Directive 89/109 of 21 December 1988. Official Journal of the European Community, L40/38 of 11 February, 1989

Part IV
Needs and Prospects of Intake Studies

CHAPTER 21

WHO International Co-operation in Exposure Studies

H. Galal-Gorchev[1]

In order to encourage international co-operation in exposure studies, Guidelines for the Study of Dietary Intake of Chemical Contaminants have been prepared by the Joint UNEP/FAO/WHO Food Contamination Monitoring Program (GEMS/Food) in collaboration with the Joint FAO/WHO Food Standards Program and the relevant committees of the Codex Alimentarius Commission (WHO Offset Publication no 87, 1985). The basic objective of these Guidelines is to aid countries with varying resources to assess the risk of human exposure to chemical contaminants in the food supply, thus helping countries to review and amend current regulatory practices. This is achieved through the process of determining exposure of a population to chemical residues in the diet and comparing these dietary intakes with those that have been judged as acceptable through the work of JMPR and JECFA in setting ADIs or PTWIs. The Guidelines provide a detailed description of procedures and methods by which such dietary intake studies may be conducted.

The collection of valid data on the food consumption habits of a population is the most difficult problem which must be overcome before any assessment can be made of the dietary intake of a contaminant. There are two general approaches to obtaining information on the dietary habits of a population or of individuals: (a) those which involve the collection of inferred data on the movement and disappearance of foodstuffs in a region or home; and (b) those which involve the collection of direct personal data on the actual amounts of food consumed by an individual or household. A summary of the methods which have been generally used are shown in Table 21.1.

The characteristics, advantages and disadvantages of the different methods of determining food consumption data are described in detail in the Guidelines. The selection of any one method over another will depend on such factors as age, educational level, motivation of the target population and, most importantly, costs and resources available.

[1]International Programme on Chemical Safety, Division of Environmental Health, World Health Organization, CM-1211 Geneva 27, Switzerland.

Table 21.1. Methods for collecting food consumption data from population groups and individuals

Assessment	Method
Individual	Food diary, weighed intake
	Duplicate portion studies
	Dietary recall
	Food frequency
Population	Food diary, weighed intake
	Dietary recall
	Food frequency
	Food disappearance methods
	household
	national

There are three approaches which can be adopted in estimating the daily intake of a contaminant based on food consumption data:

1. Total diet (i.e. market basket) studies
2. Selective studies of individual foodstuffs
3. Duplicate portion studies

The strengths and limitations of each approach are described in the Guidelines. A preferred or recommended approach for governments to adopt is not specified since the choice of which method to adopt will depend on the objectives of the assessment and the resources available.

The Guidelines have encouraged many national institutions to initiate contaminant dietary intake studies and, to a certain extent, have harmonized various aspects of such studies. GEMS/Food has co-operated with national institutions in Guatemala, Thailand and China in developing protocols and implementing intake studies.

GEMS/Food has promoted international co-operation in exposure predictions through the publication of the Guidelines for Predicting Dietary Intake of Pesticide Residues [1] and follow-up activities. The Guidelines will assist national authorities to reach a conclusion as to the acceptability of Codex MRLs from a public health point of view.

The three-tier approach to predicting pesticide residue intake proposed in the Guidelines is outlined in Fig. 21.1. TMDI (Theoretical Maximum Daily Intake) and EMDI (Estimated Maximum Daily Intake) may be estimated at either the national or international level, while the EDI (Estimated Daily Intake) can be estimated only at the national level by those who have adequate information on food consumption, the use of a given pesticide locally, and the nature and the amount of imported food.

Nine "cultural" diets have been developed using the most recent FAO Food Balance Sheets (Appendix 1). These nine different types of diet are: African, cereal-based; African, root and tuber-based; North African; Central American; South American; Chinese; Far Eastern; Eastern Mediterranean; and European.

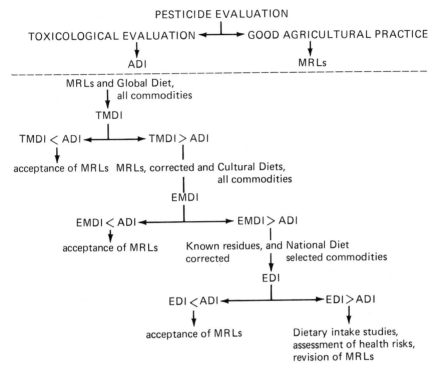

PESTICIDE EVALUATION

TOXICOLOGICAL EVALUATION ←——→ GOOD AGRICULTURAL PRACTICE

ADI   MRLs

- -

MRLs and Global Diet,
all commodities

TMDI

TMDI < ADI ←——→ TMDI > ADI

acceptance of MRLs   MRLs, corrected and Cultural Diets,
all commodities

EMDI

EMDI < ADI ←——→ EMDI > ADI

acceptance of MRLs   Known residues, and National Diet
corrected   selected commodities

EDI

EDI < ADI ←——→ EDI > ADI

acceptance of MRLs   Dietary intake studies,
assessment of health risks,
revision of MRLs

Figure 21.1. The three tier approach to predicting pesticide residue intake.

These diets are not necessarily geographical in nature but are instead based on similarities in dietary patterns. For instance, the Chinese-type diet includes not only China but Vietnam as well, and the European-type diet includes Australia, Canada, New Zealand and the USA in addition to European countries. The cultural diets are used for calculating Estimated Maximum Daily Intakes (EMDIs).

A "global" diet has been developed based on the nine cultural diets, and this global diet has been used for estimating Theoretical Maximum Daily Intakes (TMDIs). The global diet was calculated using the highest average food consumption value for individual commodities from each cultural diet. The total consumption came to 3.6 kg/day and this was adjusted to a total daily consumption of 1.5 kg solid food (Appendix 21.1). At present the global diet includes consumption figures for 67 different foods/food groups.

One major problem in estimating TMDIs and EMDIs is that many of the commodities for which MRLs have been established or recommended are not listed individually in the present food consumption database. We are in the process of improving this database by obtaining food consumption data for an increased number of food commodities in order to obtain better estimates of TMDIs and EMDIs.

To illustrate the use of the Guidelines, preliminary TMDI and EMDI calculations based on the current food consumption database are given in Appendixes

21.2 and 21.3 respectively. Once again, as stressed in the Guidelines, both the TMDIs and EMDIs are exaggerated intake predictions and should serve only as screening mechanisms to eliminate the need for further consideration of the intake of a pesticide residue. It should therefore not be concluded that proposed Codex MRLs are unacceptable when the TMDI or EMDI exceed the ADI. Instead, better estimates of intake should then be made at the national level and through actual dietary intake studies. Whenever intake studies are available, they should outweigh TMDI and EMDI predictions.

Another WHO international co-operative effort in exposure study is the Human Exposure Assessment Location (HEAL) project which is being implemented by WHO and UNEP in close co-operation with national agencies and institutions. At present, Brazil, China, India, Japan, Sweden, the USA and Yugoslavia are participating in HEAL.

The primary objectives of the project are:

- To provide comparable and valid assessment of human exposures to selected environmental pollutants
- To improve, field test, harmonize and demonstrate methods for the integrated monitoring and assessment of human exposure to environmental pollutants
- To promote the assessment of human exposures to pollutants as a basis for development of environmental control strategies for the protection of public health
- To provide an overview of existing exposures of selected populations to pollutants on a regional and global basis and, if possible, observe trends in this regard
- To improve national capabilities for environmental monitoring and human exposure assessment, particularly in the developing countries

Substances at present included in HEALs are nitrogen dioxide, lead, cadmium, DDT and hexachlorobenzene. In the HEALs, the environment in terms of the air that is breathed, the water that is drunk, and the food that is eaten, is being related to human exposure. The diet is an important route of exposure to lead, cadmium, DDT and hexachlorobenzene and therefore dietary intake studies are an integral component of HEAL. Duplicate portion studies are used to determine dietary exposure of a selected number of individuals.

References

1. WHO (1989) Guidelines for predicting dietary intake of pesticide residues. WHO, Geneva.

Appendix 21.1: Cultural diets

					Regional averages (g/capita/day)						
	Africa, cereals	Africa, roots	Central America	Chinese type	Eastern Mediterranean	European type	Eastern Asian	North African	South American	Max	Global diet
Wheat	67	52	170	112	282	278	104	419	158	419	175
Rice	115	76	66	402	117	13	308	35	115	402	168
Barley						3	2	58		58	24
Maize	174	55	66	43	25	17	36	12	48	174	73
Rye						25				25	10
Oats						5				5	2
Millet	62	16			14		4	15		62	26
Sorghum	33	19			35		3	5		35	15
Potatoes	19	12	29	19	51	206	19	51	79	206	86
Cassava	48	358	15	60			34		68	358	149
Sweet potato	12	163	43	111			7		9	163	68
Other roots	5	119	39				8		14	119	50
Sugar	57	27	101	19	84	109	52	83	85	109	46
Pulses	24	25	20		15	8	11	20	14	25	10
Groundnut	6	10					2			10	4
Coconuts	5	77	24		7		25		7	77	32
Soya oil	4		6			12	3		9	12	5
Groundnut oil	2						3			3	1

(continued)

Appendix 21.1: *Continued*

	Regional averages (g/capita/day)										
	Africa, cereals	Africa, roots	Central America	Chinese type	Eastern Mediterranean	European type	Eastern Asian	North African	South American	Max	Global diet
Palmoil	3	8				8			4	8	3
Sunflower oil						8			4	8	3
Cottonseed oil	2								2	2	1
Copra oil		5							5	5	2
Rape oil						4			4	4	2
Other oils	2	2	8						8	8	3
Butter			3		6	16		6	8	16	7
Cream						10			10	10	4
Animal fat	4	2	8	2	8	42	4	8	7	42	18
Tomatoes	7	10	20		99	75	5	104	20	104	44
Onions	5		9	7	34	20	12	24	11	34	14
Other vegetables	47	71	85	150	157	171	142	74	77	171	71
Oranges	5	7	39		32	49	21	31	44	49	20
Lemons		3	13		7			5	7	13	6
Grapefruit			13						5	13	6
Banana	10	66	68		14	17	21		39	68	29
Plantain	5	68	34						40	68	28
Apples			4		22	55	8		11	55	23
Pineapple	5	12	5				11		6	12	5
Dates					25			23		25	10

Appendix 21.1: *Continued*

	Africa, cereals	Africa, roots	Central America	Chinese type	Regional averages (g/capita/day) Eastern Mediterranean	European type	Eastern Asian	North African	South American	Max	Global diet
Grapes					32	21		10	5	32	13
Other fruit	35	46	113	50	141	96	63	100	40	141	59
Fish+seafood	25	50	44	26	35	60	79	74	38	79	33
Beef	21	14	39		17	62	12	21	59	62	26
Sheep	8	7	5		24	15	2	19	5	24	10
Pork	6	6	24	34		94	28		18	94	39
Poultry	8	7	48	6	36	39	29	16	30	48	20
Other meat	6	4				5				6	2
Offals	6	3	6		7	13	4	7	7	13	5
Milk solids	15	5	32	1	35	77	12	34	28	77	32
Eggs	4	3	14	9	15	37	17	11	14	37	16
Total	862	1406	1215	1051	1375	1669	1093	1264	1123	3591	1500

Appendix 21.2: Theoretical Maximum Daily Intakes

Vamidothion	ADI=0.008 mg/kg body wt or 0.48 mg/capita			
Commodity	MRL (mg/kg)	Global diet (g/day)	TMDI (mg/day)	TMDI (%)
Cereal grains	0.2	325	0.065	35
Grapes	0.5	13	0.007	4
Peach	0.5	59	0.030[a]	16
Pome fruits	1	27	0.027	15
Rice, husked	0.2	168	0.034	18
Sugar beet	0.5	46	0.023	12
		Total	0.185	100

TMDI < ADI% ADI = 39%

Triazophos	TADI = 0.0002 mg/kg body wt or 0.012 mg/capita			
Commodity	TMRL (mg/kg)	Global diet (g/day)	TMDI (mg/day)	TMDI (%)
Banana	1	29	0.029	27
Brussels sprout	0.1	71	0.007[b]	7
Cabbages, Head	0.1	—		
Carrot	0.1	—		
Cereal grains	0.05[c]	—		
Citrus fruits	2	32	0.064	60
Coffee beans	0.05[c]	—		
Cotton seed	0.1	—		
Onion, bulb	0.05[c]	—		
Peas	0.1	—		
Pome fruits	0.2	27	0.005	5
Potato	0.05[c]	—		
Sugar beet	0.05[c]	—		
		Total	0.106	100

TMDI > ADI% TADI = 883%

[a] TMDI obtained by using global consumption of fruits other than citrus, banana, plantain, apple, pear, pineapple, date and grape, and highest MRL for any fruit in this group.
[b] TMDI obtained by using global consumption of "other vegetables" than tomato, onion, pulse, potato, cassava, sweet potato and other roots, and highest MRL for any vegetable in this group.
[c] At or about the limit of determination.

Appendix 21.3: Estimated Maximum Daily Intake (European-type Diet)

Triazophos	TADI = 0.0002 mg/kg body wt or 0.012 mg/capita					
Commodity	F (g/day)	R (mg/kg)	P	C	EMDI (mg/day)	% EMDI
Banana (pulp)	11[a]	0.1	1	1	0.0011	5
Cabbages (washed and boiled)	39[b]	0.1	1	0.5×0.5[c]	0.0010	5
Carrots (peeled)	15	0.1	1	0.2	0.003	1
Citrus fruits (pulp)	47	0.1	1	1	0.0047	23
Peas	9	0.1	1	0.5[d]	0.0005	2
Pome fruits	64	0.2	1	1	0.0128	63
				Total =	0.0203	100

EMDI > ADI % ADI = 169%

F, food consumption (g/day)

R, residue level in the edible portion of the commodity (mg/kg)

P, correction factor for commercial processing.

C, correction factor for preparation and cooking of the food.

[a]Assumes skin is 30% of weight of banana.

[b]Includes brussel sprouts and other cabbages.

[c]Assumes all cabbages are cooked.

[d]Assumes same cooking correction factor as for cabbages.

CHAPTER 22

Means of Improving the Comparability of Intake Studies

K. Louekari[1]

Introduction

Several methods are available for estimating intake of contaminants of food and each of the methods has certain merits and limitations. At present, standardized or commonly accepted methods are developing. One of the most important steps in this process has been the preparation of "guidelines for the study of dietary intakes of chemical contaminants" by WHO in 1985 [1]. In fact, intake estimation is conducted by different methods and modifications in different countries. This is reasonable to some extent, since the risk management policies and legislation also vary from country to country. However, estimates from different countries are actually not comparable due to inconsistent methodology. The necessity for making the studies more comparable even in one country is demonstrated in the Tables 22.1 and 22.2. It is obvious, that methodological differences are responsible for the majority of the differences shown in these tables. At present, it may also be the case that methodological advances made in certain studies are not recognized and discussed by other groups working in food toxicology or risk assessment, because of the lack of a common conceptual and methodological basis.

The different methods of intake estimation are not described in detail here, since they have been covered in other chapters. This chapter considers the factors which affect the comparability of intake studies. In addition, the advantages of certain technologies used in intake estimation are commented on and suggestions are made of what information should be reported about an intake study.

The aims of intake studies are different. In many studies, the intake of a food contaminant is estimated in order to compare the intake to recommendations and to facilitate the assessment of the safety of the present rate of intake. In many of these studies there is also an estimate of high intakes, for example the ninetieth percentile of the intake or the range of the intake in the study population is given.

There are also some comparisons between countries. The problem here is to find food consumption data, which would have been collected by the same

---

[1]Ministry of Social Affairs and Health, Snellmaninkatn 7-6, SF-00130 Helsinki, Finland.

Table 22.1. The average intake of lead, cadmium and mercury in Japan

Reference	Intake (µg/day)		
	Pb	Cd	Hg
Ohmomo [2]	176.0	49.0	18.4
Horiguchi [3]	151.0		
Teraoka [4]	220.0		
Kuwabara [5]	37.0	20.0	9.9
Murakami [6]	59.4	26.6	4.0
Kjellström [7]		35.0	
Kurono [8]	167.0		

method from all the countries. Also, the analytical methods and sampling are not always comparable [12,13]. In the 1970s, a well-designed comparative study was conducted, in which Swedish, Japanese and American laboratories co-operated to provide data on the exposure to cadmium from different sources and on tissue concentrations of heavy metals [7].

Long-term changes in the intake of contaminants have been studied by Travis and Etnier [14]. In that study the trend in food consumption during the period of 1920–1975 was investigated. However, in that study, it was assumed that cadmium concentration in foods remained constant over the specified time. Another calculation was made assuming that the increase of cadmium concentration in US foods has been the same as the increase in cadmium concentration of wheat as reported by Kjellström et al. [15]. Long-term changes are difficult to study since both food consumption and contaminant contents should have been measured over the whole study period and using comparable methods.

Quality of the Analytical Data on the Concentration of Heavy Metals in Food

The representative sampling of food is important, when average intakes of a population or a subgroup are studied. One reasonable approach is to collect samples in large processing units: mills, dairies, slaughterhouses and other food

Table 22.2. The average intake of lead and cadmium in the Federal Republic of Germany

Reference	Intake (µg/week)		Comments
	Pb	Cd	
Weigert [9]	1250	330	Total diet 55 foods, thousands of samples
Boppel [10]	850		Duplicate portions, 28 samples
Kampe [11]	320	89	Total diet, about 600 samples

processors etc. [16,17]. If samples are collected from local supermarkets, care should be taken, not to choose items with some local contamination of the metals in question. A not uncommon deficit of intake studies is that the design by which the representative sampling is ascertained, is not specified in the report.

The validity of the analysis of heavy metals is critical in intake studies, since the levels found in most foods are very low. The quality control in the laboratory should include analysis of international and certified reference materials. For example reference samples of the US National Bureau of Standards were analyzed in the Finnish trace element study [17] and by Slorach et al. [18]. The total diet reference material of USDA was analyzed by Kumpulainen et al. [19] in a comparative study. In his co-operative study, Kjellström [7] organized an inter-laboratory cross-check, which makes the results of several co-operating laboratories comparable. The analytical techniques can also be controlled by performing recovery and reproducibility studies as was done for example by Buchet and Lauwerys [20]. In many intake studies, either reference samples were not analyzed or the analyses used in calculation were not made by the authors of the intake studies [14,21].

Quality of Food Consumption Data

There are two basic methods of intake estimation: duplicate portion and total diet method, with many modifications of both. Duplicate portions can be true duplicates collected from individuals from households [20] or they can be duplicates, composed in the laboratory according to statistical [18] or individual [22] food consumption data. Some of the advantages of the duplicate portions method are achieved by using the later modifications. The total diet method is often referred as the market basket method. In a market basket study purchased food samples are divided into food groups, on the basis of food consumption statistics [19,23]. Because only the homogenates of each food group are analyzed, a part of the costs of analysis is saved as compared to the situation, where more than 300 food samples are analyzed for their heavy metal content [17,24]. In another version of a total diet study, an already existing food composition data bank is used. The data bank may contain the heavy metal data of hundreds or thousands of food items [21,25]. When the data on food contaminants are already available, special emphasis can be given to the adequate design of the food consumption study.

Food balance sheets are sometimes used for estimation of intake. Their advantage is that food balances are made in a similar way in every country and consequently, their use enables comparisons between countries. However, food balance sheets do not provide information on the variation of food consumption, and the number of foods included in balance sheets is rather small. They usually cover about 100 foods, as in household surveys the consumption of 300–400 food items is recorded. Methodological differences between food balance sheets and household surveys have been elucidated by FAO [26]. When the sources of food consumption data are methodologically different in two intake studies, the results are not comparable.

Food consumption data are in most cases nationally representative. The sources of those data are often national statistics published for example by the US Department of Agriculture or Ministry of Agriculture and Fisheries in Belgium. There are also studies concerning special subgroups of the population. The lead intake of children has been studied by carefully estimating their food consumption and combining these data with the analytical concentrations of lead in foods [21,27,28]. The intake of cadmium in a heavily polluted area in the UK was studied by analyzing the content of heavy metals in local foods and the food consumption of people living in that district [29].

Estimation Phase

When food consumption data and heavy metal content data are available, an estimation of intake can be made. The problem of how to combine these sets of data has to be considered. When either (a) the food items which are analyzed are specially selected to be the same as in food consumption study or (b) when the nomenclature of a food consumption study is made according to a food composition data bank, which already exists, there should be no problem. However, in most cases, some assumption about the suitability has to be made when combining the two sets of data. These assumptions might be, for example, that the metal content of a certain food item is the same as the average of that group, or that the composition of foodstuffs like pineapple or cocoa can be taken from the tables of another country. Furthermore, an assumption has to be made, when metal contents, which were under the limit of detection, are included in the file. The way in which these results are expressed for calculation affects the estimate. In some cases these results are expressed as being at the limit of detection [29] and sometimes it is assumed that the true value is half of the limit of detection [17].

In most studies, some estimate of potential or maximal intake is given. In the Belgian report the potential intake, which is about four times the average, is calculated assuming that the concentration of lead and cadmium in foods are equal to the regulatory limit value [24]. In the studies, in which the individual food intake is recorded or duplicate portions analyzed, the range of estimated intakes gives some information concerning the highest actual intakes in the population [21]. When these studies are designed, attention should be paid to long-term exposure, and not to day-to-day variation in food consumption and intake. Also percentiles of 90, 95 or 99 are useful when the variation of intake and the possible risk groups are considered [20].

The method used when estimating contaminant intakes can affect the result in several ways. The advantages and disadvantages of different methods have been considered for example by Coomes et al. [29]. In diary studies the food consumption data can be combined with data on heavy metal concentrations in particular foods; vegetables for lead, fish for mercury etc. and consumption of these foods is recorded by the subjects. The advantage of diary studies is that they are individual and recording can be centered on those foods which are particularly interesting in respect of the specific contaminant. The main source of error in this method is that the level of the components in all the foods is often difficult to measure accurately. The advantage of the duplicate portion method is that the samples to be analyzed are ideally exact replicates of the food consumed. However, the participants do not always correctly divide the meals between themselves and the "duplicate plate." Another advantage is that in duplicate portions, the effect of food preparation on the content of additives and contaminants is included. The concentration of lead and cadmium in vegetables and fruits is decreased by processing, whereas the concentration of some toxic metals in sugar and canned foods seems to be elevated during processing as compared to raw products.

There also seem to be some basic differences between the calculation methods and duplicate portion method. Without exception in all studies, where these methods are compared the duplicate portion method results in lower estimates [18,22,24,29]. Some of the reasons for this difference have been specified above. Theoretically a well-designed duplicative portion study, consisting of a sufficient number of samples, should provide more reliable results, but actually it is not always possible to judge whether the lower estimates provided by duplicate portions studies are more valid than the other estimates.

References

1. WHO (1985) Guidelines for the study of dietary intakes of chemical contaminants, GEMS: Global Environment Monitoring System. WHO Offset Publication No. 87, Geneva
2. Ohmomo Y, Sumiya M (1982) Estimation on heavy metal intake from agricultural products. In: Kitagishi K, Heavy metal pollution in soils of Japan, pp 236–244
3. Horiguchi S, Teramoto K, Kurono T, Ninomiya K (1978) The arsenic, copper, lead, manganese and zinc contents of daily foods and beverages in Japan and the estimate of their daily intake. Osaka City Med J 24:131–141
4. Teraoka H, Morii F, Kobayashi J (1981) The concentration of 24 elements in foodstuffs and the estimation of their daily intake. Eiyo to Shokuryo 34:221–239
5. Kuwabara K, Murakami Y, Maeda K et al. (1982) Daily intake of environmental contaminants by the total diet study method in Osaka (IV). Shokuhin Eisei Hen 13:29–32
6. Murakami Y, Kuwabara K, Matsumoto M et al. (1983) Daily intake of environmental contaminants by the total diet study method in Osaka (V). Shokuhin Eisei Hen 14:59–64
7. Kjellström T (1979) Exposure and accumulation of cadmium in populations from Japan, the United States, and Sweden. Environ Health Perspect 28:169–197
8. Kurono T (1983) Lead content in food in Japan in the early 1980's with the estimation of its daily intake. Osaka City Med J 29:15–41
9. Weigert P, Muller J, Klein H, Zufelde K, Hillebrandt J (1984) Arsen, Blei, Cadmium und Quecksilber in und auf Lebensmitteln. ZEBS-hefte 1
10. Boppel B (1975) Bleigehalte vonLebensmittel. 3Blei-Aufnahme durch dietägliche Nahrung. Z Lebensm Unters Forsch 158:287–290
11. Kampe W (1983) Lead and cadmium in vegetable. Wissenschaft und Umweltl
12. Louekari K, Salminen S (1983) Intake of heavy metals in Finland, West Germany, and Japan, Food Additives and Contaminants 3:355–362

13. Horiguchi S, Teramoto K, Kurono T, Ninomiya K (1978) An attempt at comparative estimate of daily intake of several metals (As, Cu, Pb, Mn, Zn) from foods in thirty countries in the world. Osaka City Med J 24:237–242

14. Travis CC, Etnier EL (1982) Dietary intake of cadmium in the United States: 1920–1975. Environ Res 27:1–9

15. Kjellström T, Lind B, Linnman L, Elinder C (1975) Variation of cadmium concentration in Swedish wheat and barley. Arch Environ Health 30:321–328

16. Dabeka RW, McKentzie AD (1988) Lead and cadmium levels in commercial infant foods and dietary intake by infants 0–1 year old. Food Additives and Contaminants 5:333–342

17. Koivistoinen P (ed) (1980) Mineral element composition of Finnish foods. Acta Agric Scand Suppl 22

18. Slorach S, Gustafsson I-B, Jorhem L, Mattson P (1983) Intake of lead, cadmium and certain other metals via a typical Swedish weekly diet. Vår föda Suppl 1

19. Kumpulainen J, Mutanen M, Paakki M, Lehto J (1987) Validity of calculation method in estimating mineral element content of a pooled total daily diet as tested by chemical analysis. Vår Föda Suppl 1:75–82

20. Buchet JP, Lauwerys R (1983) Oral daily intake of cadmium, lead, manganese, copper, chromium, mercury, calcium, zinc and arsenic in Belgium: a duplicate meal study. Food Chem Toxic 21:19–24

21. Bander L, Morgan K, Zabik M (1983) Dietary lead intake of preschool children. Am J Public Health 73:789–794

22. Louekari K, Jolkkonen L, Varo P (1988) Exposure to cadmium from foods, estimated by analysis and calculation – comparison of methods. Food Additives Contaminants 5:111–117

23. de Vos RH, van Dokkum, Olthof PDA, Quirijns JK, Muys T, van der Poll JM (1984) Pesticides and other chemical residues in Dutch total diet samples (June 1976–July 1978). Food Chem Toxic 22:11–21

24. State Supervisory Public Health Service (1983) Surveillance program "Man and Nutrition." Rapporten 10 Hague

25. Louekari K, Uusitalo U, Pietinen P (1989) Variation and modifying factors of the exposure to lead and cadmium based on an epidemiological study. The Science of the Total Environment 84:1–12

26. FAO (1983) A comparative study of food consumption data from food balance sheets and household surveys. FAO Economic and Social Development Paper, Statistics Division, Rome

27. Sherlock JC, Barltrop D, Evans WH, Quinn MJ, Smart GA, Strehlow C (1985) Blood lead concentrations and lead intake in children of different ethnic origin. Human Toxicol 4:513–519

28. Mykkänen H, Räsänen L, Ahola M, Kimppa S (1986) Dietary intakes of mercury, lead, cadmium and arsenic by Finnish children. Human Nutr Appl Nutr 40A:32–39

29. Coomes TJ, Sherlock JC, Walters B (1982) Studies in dietary intake and extreme consumption. R Soc Health J 102:119–123

CHAPTER 23

Future Trends and Co-operation Concerning Intake Studies

S.A. Slorach[1]

Introduction

Data on the intake of foods and food constituents (nutrients, contaminants, additives, etc.) are needed to:

- Estimate health risks from food constituents as a basis for recommendations on dietary habits
- Carry out epidemiological studies on the relation between dietary components and health
- Study time-trends in dietary intakes and thus obtain an early warning of impending problems
- Set maximum permitted levels for additives and contaminants in foods

Although it is of interest to know the average intake of food constituents by the general population, from the health point of view it is much more important to obtain data on the intake by groups which are at greater risk because they have extremely low or high intakes or because they are especially sensitive due to, for example, age, pregnancy or disease. In the case of methylmercury, for example, the intake by pregnant women who consume relatively large amounts of certain fish species which contain high levels of methylmercury (e.g. pike and shark) is much more important than the intake by the "average consumer."

Quality Assurance

In recent years increasing emphasis has been placed on assuring the quality of the data produced in dietary intake studies. This includes the development and use of improved procedures for the recording, handling and verification of data col-

[1]Food Research Department, National Food Administration, Box 622, S-751 26 Uppsala, Sweden.

lected in food consumption studies. NORFOODS, EUROFOODS and INFOODS have been working for many years to improve the quality of nutrient databases.

Preanalytical and analytical quality assurance should form an integral part of any study of dietary intakes. The application of established guidelines on good laboratory practice, the analysis of standard reference materials, e.g. those available from the Community Bureau of Reference (BCR) and the National Institute of Standards and Technology (NIST), and participation in national and international intercalibration studies should help to improve the quality of the analytical data generated. There is a need to develop further certified standard reference materials covering a wider range of substances, levels and food matrices. Laboratories should be encouraged to participate in intercalibration exercises, such as those being run on aflatoxins, heavy metals and organochlorine compounds as part of the Joint UNEP/FAO/WHO Food Contamination Monitoring Programme and those run by national authorities responsible for food control or laboratory approval. Scientific journals should require that information on quality assurance procedures and results be presented together with the results of intake studies.

International Collaboration in the Development of Methodology

Dietary intake studies are time-consuming and expensive. Thus there is much to be gained by international collaboration in the development and evaluation of methods to estimate such intake. An example of this are the guidelines for predicting dietary intake of pesticide residues prepared by the Joint UNEP/ FAO/WHO Food Contamination Monitoring Programme in collaboration with the Codex Committee on Pesticide Residues [1]. These provide excellent advice on different methods of estimating pesticide residue intake. A working group within the Codex Committee on Food Additives and Contaminants, chaired by Professor Fondu, has developed guidelines for estimating food additive intake.

Methods for integrated exposure monitoring are being developed and tested within the UNEP/WHO Human Exposure Assessment Location (HEAL) Project. Sweden has co-ordinated a pilot project in which human exposure to lead and cadmium via the diet and inhaled air has been determined, together with blood levels and fecal excretion of these metals [2]. Extensive quality assurance was carried out as an integral part of the project. Dietary intake was estimated by analyzing duplicate portions of all the foods and beverages consumed by the subjects during seven consecutive 24-hour periods. The study was carried out on groups of non-smoking women in China, Japan, Yugoslavia and Sweden. In the Swedish part of the study mean daily dietary lead and cadmium intakes by the 15 subjects were 26 µg and 8.5 µg, respectively. The ratio between the highest and lowest weekly lead intakes (280 and 90 µg) was approximately three, whereas the ratio between the highest and lowest daily lead intakes (130 and 4.4 µg) was about 30. For these two metals the weekly, rather than the daily, intake is of prime interest.

International collaboration in the development and evaluation of analytical methodology is already well established, e.g. via various FAO/WHO Codex Alimentarius Committees, the AOAC, the Nordic Committee on Food Analysis and BCR. The Nordic countries have a long-standing collaboration in the development and evaluation of methods for studying food consumption. This is carried out with support from the Nordic Council of Ministers.

Many countries, especially developing countries, do not have the trained manpower and technical resources to be able to carry out dietary intake studies, but they do have serious food contamination problems. For example, exposure to pesticide residues is often very much higher in developing countries than in Western Europe and North America. Providing advice on methodology, training in analytical techniques and the necessary equipment, chemicals, etc., will enable some of these countries to carry out intake studies. The results of these investigations may well be of interest not only to the country concerned but also internationally.

Dioxin Analysis

Polychlorinated dibenzofurans (PCDFs) and polychlorinated dibenzo-p-dioxins (PCDDs) are extremely toxic substances which are present at very low picogram per gram) levels in certain foods, including human milk. For the general population the diet is the main route of exposure. Although great advances have been made in the last few years in methods to detect and quantitate these substances in foods, it is still difficult to obtain reliable data on dietary intake. One of the major problems is that the levels of PCDDs and PCDFs present in most staple foods, especially vegetable foodstuffs, are at or below the limit of quantitation with current methodology. We have recently attempted to estimate the dietary intake in Sweden by analyzing market basket samples. Unfortunately, the levels of PCDDs and PCDFs in the samples were nearly all at or below the limit of determination. Depending on whether one assumes that the levels below the limit of determination are zero, the same as the limit of determination or somewhere between these values, the estimated weekly intake will vary from 10 to 18 000 pg TCDD equivalents! International agreement on how to treat data on levels below the limit of determination when estimating dietary intakes could help to avoid a lot of confusion and misunderstanding.

There is a further problem in reporting the results of PCDD and PCDF analysis. In order to be able to carry out a toxicological evaluation of the results, it is desirable to calculate PCDD/PCDF levels in foods in terms of 2,3,7,8-TCDD-equivalents (2,3,7,8-TCDD = 2,3,7,8-tetrachlorodibenzo-p-dioxin, the most toxic substance in the group). Unfortunately, there is not yet international agreement on the various weighting factors ("TCDD equivalents") to be used when making such calculations. Thus, as shown in a report by a Nordic expert group on dioxins, when expressed as TCDD equivalents the results of a single analysis of, for example, a fish sample for PCDDs and PCDFs will vary depending on whether one uses the weighting factors proposed by the US EPA, the Nordic expert group or other authors or authorities [3]. It is to be hoped that international agreement on this subject will be reached in the near future.

Sample Banks for Future Studies

Developments in analytical methodology enable us to detect and identify hitherto unidentified substances and to quantify much lower levels than was previously possible. In order to be able to study time-trends in levels of contaminants and other food constituents and thereby trends in dietary intake and human exposure to substances not previously studied, it is necessary to establish and maintain "sample banks" containing staple foods (or market basket samples) and/or human tissues and body fluids. Such banks are being established in more and more countries, albeit often on a small scale initially.

An example of the value of such banks is provided by the recent report from Norén [4] from the Karolinska Institute in Stockholm who analyzed samples of human milk collected from 1972 to 1985. She has shown that the levels of PCDDs/PCDFs in the fat of banked human milk from the Human Milk Centre in Stockholm have decreased from about 34 pg TCDD equiv/g in 1972 to 17 pg TCDD equiv/g in 1984–85.

New Areas for Dietary Intake Studies

Up to now most studies on dietary intakes of food components have been concerned with either nutrients, contaminants or food additives. In the future the following areas will probably receive increased attention in dietary intake studies:

- Natural, non-nutrient components which have a protective effect against disease (e.g. carotenoids and indole derivatives) or pharmacological effects (e.g. monoamines) or which are of health interest for other reasons (e.g. metabolic intermediates)
- As yet unidentified toxic organohalogen compounds present in complex mixtures currently determined as EOCl, etc.
- Speciation of metals instead of determination of total lead, cadmium, etc.

International Data Exchange

Because intake studies are very time-consuming and expensive it is important to make the best possible use of the data generated. Thus international exchange and pooling of information on the composition of foods, e.g. the levels of nutrients and contaminants, is to be encouraged. In this connection it can be mentioned that NORFOODS, EUROFOODS and INFOODS are co-ordinating the exchange of data on food consumption.

The Nordic countries are pooling their data on pesticide residues and other contaminants in foods in their work on harmonization of legislation on food contaminants. Data collected in the Joint UNEP/FAO/WHO Food Contamination Monitoring Programme are being used in the Codex Alimentarius work on setting international guideline levels for heavy metals in foods.

The food industry and trade should make available the data they have on the levels of additives in the products they manufacture and sell and on the consumption of their products by different population groups. This would facilitate reliable estimation of the dietary intake of such additives and avoid unnecessary duplication of effort.

References

1. WHO (1989) Guidelines for predicting dietary intake of pesticide residues. Report prepared by the Joint UNEP/FAO/WHO Food Contamination Monitoring Programme in collaboration with the Codex Committee on Pesticide Residues, World Health Organization, Geneva
2. Vahter M, Slorach SA (1990) Exposure monitoring of lead and cadmium. An international pilot study within the WHO/UNEP Human Exposure Assessment Location (HEAL) Programme United Nations Environment Programme. Nairobi
3. Nordisk dioxinriskbedömning (Nordic evaluation of health risks from dioxin) (1988) Report from a Nordic expert group. Nordic Council of Ministers report NORD 1988: 49, Copenhagen
4. Norén K (1988) Changes in the levels of organochlorine pesticides, polychlorinated biphenyls, dibenzo-*p*-dioxins and dibenzofurans in human milk from Stockholm 1972–1985. Chemosphere 17:39–49

CHAPTER 24

Dietary Intakes: Summary and Perspectives

R. Kroes[1]

The aim of this volume was to bring together nutritionists and toxicologists from academia, industry and government to discuss the current problems and possible perspectives related to dietary surveys. In addition the relevance of dietary intake data to the assurance of health and safety has been addressed.

The various chapters have indicated that nutritionists are very creative in designing dietary surveys. Each type of survey has its merits and different approaches answer different questions. Two main drawbacks of dietary survey methods have been identified: with retrospective methods insufficient memory may confuse the results whereas with prospective methods there may be changes in intake during recording. In addition, the within-person variability may also influence the results. More emphasis needs to be focused on improvements in both retrospective and prospective studies and new approaches may be necessary to overcome current problems in their design.

However, this should not prevent the urgent development of methods for the co-ordination and where possible the harmonization of methods and most importantly the standardization of the presentation of results.

International collaboration, as for example the GEMS/FOOD program of the WHO, should be encouraged. At the same time those countries which are currently carrying out dietary surveys should collaborate as much as possible in order to gain agreement. Methods should be well described and justification given for the methodologies used.

Comparability between methods should be investigated and improved. When market basket studies and duplicate diet studies are carried out in the same region the results are surprisingly comparable. Dietary surveys may provide information about differences in intake within a region or country or about differences between countries. In addition they provide information on food consumption and may show how food habits change in the course of time due to cultural changes or public campaigns. In the future, dietary surveys should also provide

[1]National Institute of Public Health and Environmental Protection, P.O. Box 1, 3720 BA Bilthoven, The Netherlands.

means for forecasting dietary changes, dietary habits and consumption patterns. In this endeavor comparability, standardization and validation will be important keywords.

Dietary surveys not only provide information on food habits and trends in food consumption, they also provide data on the actual intake of macro- and micro-nutrients, food additives and contaminants. Such data may well be used for epidemiological studies and it seems worth while to establish databanks and sample banks for biomonitoring.

When comparing intakes with RDAs it is important to consider the bioavailability of the substances concerned. There is a need for the establishment of generally recognized RDAs or ranges of RDAs. This would allow the RDAs to be used as a yardstick for comparison with national intake data, in order to investigate the need for public campaigns and the fortification of food components or to advise on supplementation.

Dietary surveys also provide data on the actual intake of food additives and contaminants. This is a very important issue – not necessarily because of a real risk but certainly because of the public concern involved: chemophobia has been the disease of the eighties. It is apparent that there is a need for appropriate validated and quality controlled analytical methods which are comparable with each other. These standardized methods could then be used not only to determine actual intakes but also for control measures.

It has been shown that actual intakes of food additives and contaminants are in general well below the ADI: intakes of pesticides and veterinary drug residues are around 1% of the ADI; aspartame is consumed at about one-twentieth of the ADI. This suggests that more accurate data on these types of additives and contaminants are not needed as data indicate the absence of real risk. This would allow attention to be focused on naturally occurring toxoids, such as aflatoxin, persistent chemicals and radionuclides. However, it may be necessary to develop more accurate data on the intake of additives and contaminants to present to the general public in order to show that current chemophobia is not justified and focused on the wrong substances.

But how should such data be presented to the general public? How should risk be communicated? How can public perceptions be changed? There needs to be a multidisciplinary approach in which nutritionists, toxicologists and epidemiologists are joined by sociologists and social psychologists. In such an approach more attention should be devoted to the identification of certain risks, or the absence of risks, in groups of the population. A further aspect is the need to improve methods for calculating potential intakes. A working group needs to be initiated to investigate this specific problem.

This summary has only covered some of the points raised in earlier chapters. The topics which have been raised now need to be followed up.

Index

DATE DUE

NOV 1 1 1991			
FEB 1 0 1994			
JUN 1 1 1997			
JUN 1 1 1997			
JUL 1 8 2005			
APR 0 3 2011			